Orthobiologic Concepts in Foot and Ankle

Guest Editor

STUART D. MILLER, MD

FOOT AND ANKLE CLINICS

www.foot.theclinics.com

Consulting Editor
MARK S. MYERSON, MD

December 2010 • Volume 15 • Number 4

SAUNDERS an imprint of ELSEVIER, Inc.

W.B. SAUNDERS COMPANY
A Division of Elsevier Inc.

1600 John F. Kennedy Blvd. ● Suite 1800 ● Philadelphia, PA 19103-2899

http://www.theclinics.com

FOOT AND ANKLE CLINICS Volume 15, Number 4
December 2010 ISSN 1083-7515, ISBN-13: 978-1-4377-2451-6

Editor: Debora Dellapena
Developmental Editor: Donald Mumford

Foot and Ankle Clinics (ISSN 1083-7515) is published quarterly by Elsevier, Inc., 360 Park Avenue South, New York, NY 10010-1710. Months of issue are March, June, September, and December. Periodicals postage paid at New York, NY, and additional mailing offices. Subscription price per year is $271.00 (US individuals), $357.00 (US institutions), $134.00 (US students), $308.00 (Canadian individuals), $422.00 (Canadian institutions), $184.00 (Canadian students), $397.00 (foreign individuals), $422.00 (foreign institutions), and $184.00 (foreign students). To receive student/resident rate, orders must be accompanied by name of affiliated institution, date of term, and the *signature* of program/residency coordinator on institution letterhead. Orders will be billed at individual rate until proof of status is received. Foreign air speed delivery is included in all *Clinics* subscription prices. All prices are subject to change without notice. **POSTMASTER:** Send address changes to *Foot and Ankle Clinics*, Elsevier Health Sciences Division, Subscription Customer Service, 3251 Riverport Lane, Maryland Heights, MO 63043. **Customer Service: 1-800-654-2452 (US and Canada). From outside of the United States and Canada, call 314-447-8871. Fax: 314-447-8029. E-mail: JournalsCustomerService-usa@elsevier.com (for print support); JournalsOnlineSupport-usa@elsevier.com (for online support).**

Reprints. For copies of 100 or more, of articles in this publication, please contact the Commercial Reprints Department, Elsevier Inc., 360 Park Avenue South, New York, NY 10010-1710. Tel.: 212-633-3812; Fax: 212-462-1935; E-mail: reprints@elsevier.com.

Printed and bound in the United Kingdom
Transferred to Digital Print 2011

Contributors

CONSULTING EDITOR

MARK S. MYERSON, MD
Director, Institute for Foot and Ankle Reconstruction at Mercy, Mercy Medical Center, Baltimore, Maryland

GUEST EDITOR

STUART D. MILLER, MD
Attending Surgeon, Department of Orthopaedic Surgery, Union Memorial Hospital, Baltimore, Maryland

AUTHORS

ANSWORTH A. ALLEN, MD
Associate Attending Orthopaedic Surgeon, Department of Orthopaedic Surgery, The Hospital for Special Surgery; Associate Professor of Clinical Orthopaedic Surgery, Weill Cornell Medical College, New York, New York

CHRISTOPHER BIBBO, DO, DPM, FACS, FACFAS
Chief, Foot and Ankle Section, Department of Orthopaedics, Marshfield Clinic, Marshfield, Wisconsin

ANGELO CACCHIO, MD
Department of Physical Medicine and Rehabilitation, University of Rome, Rome, Italy

CHRISTOPHER W. DIGIOVANNI, MD
Professor and Chief, Division of Foot and Ankle Surgery; Program Director, Department of Orthopaedic Surgery, The Warren Alpert School of Medicine at Brown University, Rhode Island Hospital, Providence, Rhode Island

HARALAMPOS T. DINOPOULOS, MD
Trauma Fellow, Academic Department of Trauma and Orthopedic Surgery, University of Leeds, United Kingdom

SAADIQ F. EL-AMIN, MD, PhD
Assistant Professor, Division of Orthopaedic Surgery, Southern Illinois University School of Medicine; Adjunct Assistant Professor, Department of Computer and Electrical Engineering/Biomedical Engineering Program, Department of Medical Microbiology, Immunology and Cell Biology, Southern Illinois University School of Medicine, Springfield, Illinois

JORGE FILIPPI, MD
Assistant Professor, Department of Orthopedic Surgery, Pontifical Catholic University of Chile, Santiago, Chile

JOHN P. FURIA, MD
SUN Orthopedics and Sports Medicine, Department of Orthopedic Surgery, Lewisburg, Pennsylvania

PETER V. GIANNOUDIS, MB, MD, FRCS
Professor, Department of Trauma and Orthopedic Surgery, University of Leeds; Professor, Academic Orthopedic Unit, Leeds General Infirmary University Hospital, Leeds, United Kingdom

GREGORY P. GUYTON, MD
Greater Chesapeake Orthopaedic Associates; Department of Orthopaedic Surgery, Union Memorial Hospital, Baltimore, Maryland

P. SHAWN HATFIELD, DPM
Podiatry Associates of Indiana, Indianapolis, Indiana

BRYAN J. HAWKINS, MD
Central States Ortho Specialists Inc, Tulsa, Oklahoma

ANDREW HIGGS, MBBS, FRACS
Fellow in Foot and Ankle Surgery, Avon Orthopaedic Centre, Southmead Hospital, Bristol, United Kingdom

JONATHAN HINDS, BS
University Medical and Dental School of New Jersey, New Brunswick, New Jersey

MACALUS V. HOGAN, MD
Senior Orthopaedic Resident, Academic Orthopaedic Training Program, Department of Orthopaedic Surgery, University of Virginia, Charlottesville, Virginia

CATO T. LAURENCIN, MD, PhD
Professor, Department of Orthopedic Surgery, The University of Connecticut School of Medicine, University of Connecticut Health Center, Farmington; Professor, Department of Chemical, Materials and Biomolecular Engineering, The University of Connecticut, Storrs, Connecticut

NICOLA MAFFULLI, MD, MS, PhD, FRCS(Orth), FFSEM(UK)
Centre for Sports and Exercise Medicine, Department of Orthopedics, Barts and the London School of Medicine and Dentistry, London, Great Britain, United Kingdom

STUART D. MILLER, MD
Attending Surgeon, Department of Orthopaedic Surgery, Union Memorial Hospital, Baltimore, Maryland

MARK S. MYERSON, MD
Director, Institute for Foot and Ankle Reconstruction at Mercy, Mercy Medical Center, Baltimore Maryland

VINOD K. PANCHBHAVI, MD, FRCS (Eng), FACS
Professor of Orthopedic Surgery; Chief, Division of Foot and Ankle Surgery, Department of Orthopedic Surgery, University of Texas Medical Branch, Galveston, Texas

JAMES M. PETRICEK, MSE, MBA
BioMimetic Therapeutics, Inc, Franklin, Tennessee

JAN D. ROMPE, MD
OrthoTrauma Evaluation Center, Department of Orthopedics, Mainz, Germany

IAN G. WINSON, MBChB, FRCS
Consultant Orthopaedic Surgeon, Avon Orthopaedic Centre, Southmead Hospital, Bristol, United Kingdom

Contents

Preface: Orthobiologic Concepts in Foot and Ankle   xi

Stuart D. Miller

The Indications and Use of Bone Morphogenetic Proteins in Foot, Ankle, and Tibia Surgery   543

Saadiq F. El-Amin, MaCalus V. Hogan, Answorth A. Allen, Jonathan Hinds, and Cato T. Laurencin

Tissue engineering is an area of rapid growth. Tissue engineering in orthopedic surgery involves the use of growth factors, mesenchymal stem cells, and scaffolds, individually or in combination, toward the growth and restoration of various musculoskeletal tissues, such as ligaments, tendons, muscles, nerves, and bone. These advances are constantly evolving in foot and ankle surgery as well. Bone morphogenetic proteins (BMPs) have played an integral role in the advancement of tissue engineering strategies across multiple orthopedic subspecialities and have proved to play a role in the development of bone and musculoskeletal tissues. BMPs have recently been applied in several areas of foot and ankle surgery, including acute fracture augmentation, nonunions, and arthrodesis, with promising results. This article reviews the key aspects of clinical translation of strategies in tissue engineering as well as current applications and results of BMP use in tibia, foot, and ankle surgery. Future applications of BMP and novel materials in foot and ankle surgery are also reviewed.

The Use of Proximal and Distal Tibial Bone Graft in Foot and Ankle Procedures   553

Ian G. Winson and Andrew Higgs

The techniques of proximal and distal tibial bone grafting have been well described in the literature. With the growth of a variety of new bone grafting techniques, the proximal and distal tibial bone sites remain reliable and safe for the retrieval of cancellous graft. These sites, particularly the upper tibia, provide large amounts of cancellous graft with little donor site morbidity. Proximal and distal tibial bone grafting remains a technique against which other grafting techniques should be measured.

Synthetic Bone Grafting in Foot and Ankle Surgery   559

Vinod K. Panchbhavi

Synthetic bone graft materials have an established role as osteoconductive materials. The basic function is providing a matrix to support the attachment of bone-forming cells for subsequent bone formation, but these materials in various forms can be used for other functions. They can be used as a vehicle for local antibiotic delivery and in injectable form they can be used in a minimally invasive fashion to fill voids and strengthen purchase of screws in osteoporotic bones. They can provide prolonged structural support, which is important for early weight bearing in the lower extremity. These are some of the qualities that may not be obtained from autograft bone, the traditional gold standard for bone grafting. Therefore, these synthetic bone graft substitutes have earned a unique place in the armamentarium when issues such as bone defect, bone quality, and bone infection challenge bone healing and repair. This article reviews the basic science and use of such materials in foot and ankle surgery for conditions related to trauma, tumors, and infection.

Biologics in Foot and Ankle Surgery   577

Bryan J. Hawkins

This article is another review of clinical application of the use of bone morphogenetic proteins, specifically rhBMP2 Infuse Bonegraft, in the treatment of both acute and chronic fracture and fusion situations. Overall experience is reported with particular detail to the use of biologics in the treatment of problems involving the tibia, foot, and ankle.

Autologous Bone Graft: When Shall We Add Growth Factors?   597

Peter V. Giannoudis and Haralampos T. Dinopoulos

Although the unquestionable value of autologous bone grafting and the analogous value of the reaming by-products in nonunion treatment have been mentioned extensively in the literature, there is ongoing vivid discussion for the treatment of those case scenarios where the fracture nonunion is complicated by other local environment adverse circumstances. The graft expansion with growth factors as the bone morphogenetic proteins (BMPs) offers the possibility to reduce the number of operative procedures, complications, length of hospital stay, and time to union. In this article, we consider the potential clinical scenarios for graft expansion with BMPs.

Stem Cells in Bone Grafting: Trinity Allograft with Stem Cells and Collagen/Beta-Tricalcium Phosphate with Concentrated Bone Marrow Aspirate   611

Gregory P. Guyton and Stuart D. Miller

The orthopedic foot and ankle surgeon needs bone grafts in the clinical situation of fracture healing and in bone-fusion procedures. This article briefly outlines thought processes and techniques for 2 recent options for the surgeon. The Trinity product is a unique combination of allograft bone and allograft stem cells. The beta-tricalcium phosphate and collagen materials provide an excellent scaffold for bone growth; when combined with concentrated bone marrow aspirate, they also offer osteoconductive and osteoinductive as well as osteogenerative sources for new bone formation.

The Evolution of rhPDGF-BB in Musculoskeletal Repair and its Role in Foot and Ankle Fusion Surgery   621

Christopher W. DiGiovanni and James M. Petricek

Platelet-derived growth factor (PDGF) is one of the most thoroughly studied proteins in the body. Research has progressively highlighted the role of PDGF during wound healing and in the bone repair cascade. This research has resulted in FDA approval of 2 products containing a recombinant version of the protein, rhPDGF-BB, for treating chronic diabetic foot ulcers and periodontal bone defects. This article reviews the applicable basic science and mechanisms of action of PDGF, with attention to the increasingly defined role of rhPDGF-BB in initiating bone regeneration. The most recent data from prospective clinical trials evaluating the use of rhPDGF-BB in combination with beta tricalcium phosphate as a substitute for autogenous bone graft in hindfoot and ankle arthrodesis are also summarized.

Platelet-Rich Plasma Concentrate to Augment Bone Fusion   641

Christopher Bibbo and P. Shawn Hatfield

Within the foot and ankle literature, there exists only a handful of basic science and clinical articles reporting on the efficacy and clinical utility of platelet-rich plasma (PRP). This article discusses the concept and basic science of PRP, and clinical applications of PRP for the augmentation of bone healing in foot and ankle surgery. The authors also provide a classification system that assesses relative risks for poor bone healing and the need for orthobiologic augmentation.

Shock Wave Therapy as a Treatment of Nonunions, Avascular Necrosis, and Delayed Healing of Stress Fractures   651

John P. Furia, Jan D. Rompe, Angelo Cacchio, and Nicola Maffulli

Shock wave therapy (SWT) stimulates angiogenesis and osteogenesis. SWT is commonly used to treat soft tissue musculoskeletal conditions such as fasciopathies and tendinopathies. Recent basic science and clinical data suggest that SWT can also be used to treat disorders of bone. Nonunions, avascular necrosis, and delayed healing of stress fractures have all been successfully treated with SWT. Success rates with SWT are equal to those with standard surgical treatment, but SWT has the advantage of decreased morbidity. The procedure is safe, well tolerated, yields few complications, and, typically, can be performed on an outpatient basis. SWT is a viable noninvasive alternative to stimulate healing of bone.

Bone Block Lengthening of the Proximal Interphalangeal Joint for Managing the Floppy Toe Deformity   663

Mark S. Myerson and Jorge Filippi

The short floppy toe, an iatrogenic condition in which the digit lacks structural stability, results from excessive resection of the distal aspect of the proximal phalanx during correction of claw or hammer toe deformity. The involved toe is much shorter than the adjacent digit, which it will often overlap. Little attention has been given to the cause and treatment of the floppy toe deformity in the literature. As an iatrogenic condition, the best treatment is prevention. This article discusses the various procedures for the surgical correction of the floppy toe deformity.

Index   669

FORTHCOMING ISSUES

March 2011
Nerve Problems of the Lower Extremity
John S. Gould, MD, *Guest Editor*

June 2011
Current and New Techniques for Primary
and Revision Arthrodesis
Beat Hintermann, MD, *Guest Editor*

RECENT ISSUES

September 2010
Infection, Ischemia, and Amputation
Michael S. Pinzur, MD, *Guest Editor*

June 2010
The Pediatric Foot and Ankle
Raymond J. Sullivan, MD, *Guest Editor*

March 2010
Traumatic Foot and Ankle Injuries Related
to Recent International Conflicts
Eric M. Bluman, MD, PhD,
and James R. Ficke, MD, *Guest Editors*

THE CLINICS ARE NOW AVAILABLE ONLINE!

Access your subscription at:
www.theclinics.com

Preface

Orthobiologic Concepts in Foot and Ankle

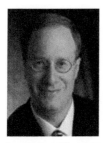

Stuart D. Miller, MD
Guest Editor

This issue of *Foot and Ankle Clinics* focuses on the complex issue of bone grafting. While orthopedic surgeons continue to evolve methods of bone fixation and fusion, the variety of bone graft, bone substitutes, and biologic augmentation has exploded. Early in my career, I left the iliac crest, believing the patients' discomfort from the graft donor site outweighed the benefits. The proximal tibia seemed an ideal source of cancellous bone and some corticocancellous grafts could also be harvested. I sometimes backfilled with allograft and sometimes with bone substitute. With better understanding of orthopedic biology, I have drifted to allograft or bone substitute, augmented by iliac crest bone marrow aspirate. I am a "stem cell believer" and use the Trinity allograft with stem cells when not autoharvesting. This circular trip included voyages to the distal tibia (one fracture ended my harvesting there) and a seemingly endless stream of the "latest and greatest" bone substitutes.

The issue hopes to help clarify individual preferences and illuminate options. We have also included the article on shock-wave influence on fracture healing, to help the surgeon realize that the answers are still unresolved. The myriad forces at work in bone healing will provide fodder for our next generation of scientists and clinicians to resolve; let's hope they not think us too silly for our choices. The choice of bone graft or substitute will always be secondary to surgical technique and skill in determining outcome and success.

Stuart D. Miller, MD
Department of Orthopaedic Surgery
Union Memorial Hospital
Baltimore, MD 21218, USA

E-mail address:
smiller@gcoa.net

Foot Ankle Clin N Am 15 (2010) xi
doi:10.1016/j.fcl.2010.09.004
1083-7515/10/$ — see front matter © 2010 Elsevier Inc. All rights reserved.

The Indications and Use of Bone Morphogenetic Proteins in Foot, Ankle, and Tibia Surgery

Saadiq F. El-Amin, MD, PhD[a,b,c], MaCalus V. Hogan, MD[d],
Answorth A. Allen, MD[e,f], Jonathan Hinds, BS[g],
Cato T. Laurencin, MD, PhD[h,i],*

KEYWORDS

- BMP • Growth factors • Tissue engineering • Foot
- Ankle • Tibia

TISSUE ENGINEERING IN FOOT AND ANKLE SURGERY

Orthopedic surgery has been influenced significantly by progress in tissue engineering, which over the last several years has made major strides in the creation of engineered tissue for potential clinical use. Tissue engineering is an interdisciplinary science that combines the basic principles of biology, chemistry, physics, and engineering to construct living tissues from their cellular components. Engineered tissue

[a] Division of Orthopaedic Surgery, Southern Illinois University School of Medicine, PO Box 19679, Springfield, IL 62794-9620, USA
[b] Department of Computer and Electrical Engineering/Biomedical Engineering Program, Southern Illinois University, Carbondale, IL 62901, USA
[c] Department of Medical Microbiology, Immunology and Cell Biology (MMICB), Southern Illinois University School of Medicine, Springfield, IL 62794-9620, USA
[d] Academic Orthopaedic Training Program, Department of Orthopaedic Surgery, University of Virginia, Box 800159, Charlottesville, VA 22908, USA
[e] Department of Orthopaedic Surgery, The Hospital for Special Surgery, 535 East 70th Street, New York, NY 10021, USA
[f] Weill Cornell Medical College, New York, NY, USA
[g] University Medical and Dental School of New Jersey-Robert Wood Johnson, 1 Robert Wood Johnson Place, New Brunswick, NJ 08901, USA
[h] Department of Orthopedic Surgery, The University of Connecticut School of Medicine, University of Connecticut Health Center, 263 Farmington Avenue, Farmington, CT 06030, USA
[i] Department of Chemical, Materials and Biomolecular Engineering, The University of Connecticut, Storrs, CT, USA
* Corresponding author. Department of Orthopedic Surgery, The University of Connecticut School of Medicine, University of Connecticut Health Center, 263 Farmington Avenue, Farmington, CT 06030.
E-mail address: laurencin@uchc.edu

Foot Ankle Clin N Am 15 (2010) 543–551
doi:10.1016/j.fcl.2010.08.001
1083-7515/10/$ – see front matter. Published by Elsevier Inc.

foot.theclinics.com

is hoped to make the augmentation or replacement of congenitally defective, impaired, injured, or otherwise damaged human tissue with synthetic biologic material possible.[1] To date, this kind of engineering has made significant advances in the design and development of biologic tissues such as the bladder, aorta, skin, breast, muscle, bone, cartilage, and tendon.[2–8] These engineered tissues have been studied in many aspects with regard to their close correlation and biocompatibility with natural tissue counterparts, biostability and integration into host material, and ultimate restoration of normal structural and functional characteristics.[1–8]

Tissue engineering is defined as the application of biologic, chemical, and engineering principles toward the repair, restoration, or regeneration of living tissues using biomaterials, cells, and other factors, alone and in combination.[9] In orthopedics, emerging treatment strategies are geared toward the improved repair and regeneration of musculoskeletal tissues. The construction of engineered bone substitutes incorporates many important design considerations to ensure the development of matrices that mimic the 3-dimensional properties of native tissue. The matrix serves as a template or scaffold material for the optimal growth of cells and new tissue formation. Ideally the material is chosen based on the intended function and use of the tissue-engineered matrix. The design considerations span from mechanical integrity to porosity.[10]

Advances in foot and ankle orthopedics have been imperative in the improvement of clinical outcomes that pertain to the treatment of fractures, repair of delayed unions and nonunions, and arthrodeses. Improvements in internal fixation, soft tissue handling, and biologic manipulation of fractures, such as use of growth factors, stem cell augmentation, electricity, and ultrasonography, have all contributed to this improvement.[11]

Soft tissue injuries and fractures of the lower extremity present issues when the natural healing process of the body is unable to occur or does not do so effectively. This process is important, especially in the case of fracture nonunions or significant traumatic bone loss, making surgical intervention to bridge the gap necessary. For bone formation to occur, certain types of cells must be present during several biologic events, such as the availability of mesenchymal stem cells and their ability to serve as osteogenic cells. In addition, the osteoconductive property of bone is important. Osteoconduction is the property by which a graft, when placed in an osseous site, functions as a scaffold for the attachment and proliferation of bone-forming cells, neovascular ingrowth, and deposition and calcification of the bone matrix. Osteoconductive agents include calcium ceramics and collagen. Commercially, there are a variety of crystalline calcium-based ceramics, including tricalcium phosphate granules, coralline hydroxyapatite, and calcium hydroxyapatite composites. Type I collagen alone is usually a poor graft substitute. To enhance neo-osteogenesis, collagen is often combined with growth factors (ie, bone morphogenetic proteins [BMPs]), progenitor cells, or other osteoinductive components.[12] Examples of calcium-based ceramics include Healos (DePuy Spine, Inc, Raynham, MA, USA), which is composed of cross-linked collagen coated with hydroxyapatite, and Collagraft (Zimmer and Collagen Corporation, Warsaw, IN, USA), which consists of a mixture of porous beads composed of 60% hydroxyapatite and 40% tricalcium phosphate ceramic and fibrillar collagen.[13]

Osteoinduction is equally important because it is the biologic stimulus that can direct and upregulate the formation of bone and migration of bone-forming cells. Osteoinductivity is the property by which the graft recruits mesenchymal stem cells and modulates their conversion to bone-forming cells to produce new bone even at extraskeletal implant sites. Osteoinductive agents include platelet gel concentrates, demineralized bone matrix, and electrical bone stimulation. The presence of growth factors, located in the alpha granules of platelets, are imperative in the induction of bone growth.[13] Lastly, osteogenesis refers to new bone formed on or around the graft by bone forming cells of graft or host origin.

In the past, improved union rates and outcomes have been attributed to increased mechanical stability afforded by the advances of fixation devices, including external fixation.[1] Moreover, the increased utility of operative intervention for complex limb salvage in entities such as Charcot neuroarthropathy has resulted in increased awareness of the complexities of bone consolidation, despite the availability and use of improved fixation constructs.[14] More recently, appreciation of the capacity of biologic modulation of the healing process has led to the proliferation of a class of substances known as orthobiologic agents, which are thought to increase the likelihood and rate of bone healing.[9]

Methods have been introduced into surgical practice to assist in the incorporation of bone grafts, either autografts or allografts, and bone graft substitutes have been developed to combat these situations in foot and ankle surgery. Autografts are considered to be most reliable for bone graft procedures because of the intrinsic osteogenic and osteoinductive properties found in the native bone. A key disadvantage of this approach is that a separate procedure is often necessary for tissue harvest from an alternate site, which is a cause of donor-site morbidity. Allografts remove the issue of donor-site morbidity but carry significant concern related to the risk of disease transmission.[15] Increased disease transmission and morbidity have begun to be alleviated with the advent of bone graft substitutes, which include demineralized bone matrix, calcium phosphate, platelet-rich plasma, and bone marrow aspirate.[16]

BMPs were first described in the literature in 1965 by Urist,[17] who observed de novo bone formation in rabbits after implantation of proteins from decalcified bone into soft tissue pouches. These proteins were then termed BMPs[18] and were subsequently found to be a part of the larger transforming growth factor β superfamily.[19] At present, there are approximately 20 BMPs, of which 7 have been proved to play prominent roles in bone formation.[20] These proteins interact with serine/threonine kinase receptors and BMP type I and type II receptors at the cell surface.[21] This interaction ultimately leads to the phosphorylation of transcription-regulating SMAD proteins, which are then translocated to the cell nucleus, leading to the expression of osteogenesis-specific genes.[22]

Recent studies have demonstrated the application of BMPs in trauma management, spinal surgery, osteonecrosis, and repair of segmental defects.[14,23] At present, recombinant human BMP (rhBMP)-2 (Infuse, Medtronic, Minneapolis, MN, USA) and rhBMP-7 are commercially available, and the US Food and Drug Administration (FDA) approved their use in posterior lumbar fusion, care of open tibial fractures, and treatment of tibial nonunions that have failed attempts at repair.[24] The clinical application of BMPs in lower-extremity surgery has evolved significantly over the past decade, with an increasing number of reports of their use in fracture treatment, arthrodesis, and nonunion repair.

Schuberth and colleagues[14] reported a retrospective review of the use of BMPs in 38 high-risk foot and ankle cases in 35 patients. All reviewed cases were considered as high risk for bone-healing complications, such as nonunion or infection. Cases varied from complex fusions and distal tibial osteotomies to repair of nonunions. Several variables that could alter the degree of healing were incorporated, including age, diagnosis of diabetes mellitus, Charcot neuroarthropathy, prior infection, type of procedure, use of femoral head allograft, electrical bone stimulation, and external fixation. The investigators observed an 84% incidence of successful bone healing and concluded that BMPs provide a stimulus for healing in complex tibia, foot, and ankle surgery. This conclusion was further supported by a prospective study that evaluated the effect of rhBMP-2 when used in high-risk ankle and hindfoot fusions.[25] The investigators reported a mean union time of 10 weeks in 45 cases when using rhBMP-2. In a recent retrospective analysis of rhBMP-2 augmentation in 112 high-risk ankle and hindfoot fusion cases in 69 patients, the investigators observed a 96% union rate, with a mean fusion time of 11 weeks and wound complications in only 3 patients. The investigators concluded that rhBMP-2 is an effective supplement for bone healing in high-risk foot and ankle fusion.[26] Kanakaris and colleagues[27] reported the use of BMP-7 in 19 fusions (including 7 in the ankle, talonavicular, or subtalar joints). They observed fair to excellent subjective outcomes in all 7 cases, with an average of 3.4 months to clinical union and an overall 90% healing rate.

The use of BMP in the care of fractures of the lower extremity has been focused in most cases on the tibia.[23,28] The prospective, controlled, randomized study by Govender and colleagues[29] evaluating the safety and efficacy of rhBMP-2 use in open tibial fractures was one of the first trials of its kind. A total of 450 patients with open tibial fractures were randomized into a control group (intramedullary nail [IMN] fixation and soft tissue care) or an IMN fixation group with rhBMP-2 (0.75 or 1.5 mg/mL) augmentation. The rhBMP-2 was delivered on a collagen sponge placed at the time of wound closure. The outcome was measured based on the number of patients requiring subsequent intervention for delayed union or nonunion within a year. With a 94% follow-up, the group that was administered 1.5 mg/mL of rhBMP-2 had a 44% reduced risk of failure, significantly faster fracture healing, and fewer hardware failures and infections than the control group. The investigators concluded that 1.5 mg/mL of rhBMP-2 was safer than and superior to IMN fixation alone for reducing the need for secondary procedures after treatment of open tibial fractures. A follow-up subgroup analysis of 2 prospective randomized trials evaluated 131 patients with Gustilo-Anderson type IIIA or IIIB open tibial fractures treated with rhBMP-2, 1.5 mg/mL, and 113 patients treated with only IMN. The rhBMP-2 subgroup showed improved outcomes, with fewer bone-grafting procedures, fewer invasive secondary interventions, and a lower infection rate. This finding further demonstrated the clinical effectiveness of rhBMP-2 use in severe open tibial fractures.[30] Another well-designed clinical study showed that BMP-2 in combination with freeze-dried allograft was found to be as safe and effective as an autograft when used for reconstruction of cortical defects after diaphyseal tibial fractures.[31] Furthermore, Ristiniemi and colleagues[32] reported that rhBMP-7 accelerated healing and shortened time away from work when used as augmentation for pilon fractures treated with external fixation. These studies further support the increasing use of BMP in tibia, foot, and ankle surgery.

The use of BMP in nonunion repair has increased over the past few decades as well. The FDA has approved recombinant human osteogenic protein-1 (rhOP-1 or BMP-7) for use in recalcitrant nonunions in long-bone fractures.[33] Johnson and colleagues[34] reported a case series of 4 patients with severe distal tibia metaphyseal nonunions. Each patient had failed an average of 5.8 surgical treatments, with an average nonunion time of 24.8 months, and was treated with debridement of fibrous tissue, sequestrectomy, deformity correction, internal fixation, and human BMP implantation. At 4.4 months, 3 of 4 patients had healed. A controlled, prospective, randomized, multicenter trial evaluating rhOP-1 showed promising results as well. In this study, 122 patients with 124 tibial nonunions were randomized into treatment groups of either IMN plus rhOP-1[1] or IMN plus autograft.[2] At 2-year follow-up, there was no statistically significant difference in outcome between the 2 groups. The investigators concluded that rhOP-1 was safe and effective for the treatment of tibial nonunions.[35] Moghaddam and colleagues[36] reported their experience with the use of BMP-7 in treating 57 atrophic long-bone nonunions in 54 patients. Of these nonunions, 26 were in the tibia. At the 6-month follow-up, there were no perioperative or postoperative complications. Bony healing was confirmed clinically and radiographically in 47 of the 57 treated nonunions. It is reasonable to assume that the use of BMP for nonunions will continue to expand as technology improves.

Complications associated with use of BMP in the lower extremity must still be delineated. A recent report on BMP-2 use in complex tibial fractures showed that patients receiving BMP-2 more frequently developed heterotopic bone, and as a result, the rate of reoperation increased.[37] This finding supports the notion that limitations to BMP use are mostly because of its relative infancy in clinical application. As with many new innovations, more well-designed larger clinical studies are needed.

FUTURE TRENDS FOR BMP APPLICATION IN FOOT AND ANKLE SURGERY

Nanotechnology and its role in tissue engineering are growing. The application of nanotechnology in orthopedic surgery has evolved as well. These developments potentially fast forward the use of BMPs in foot and ankle surgery for both bone and soft tissue applications.

Recent studies by the authors' research group have focused on polymer-based cement systems using biodegradable polyphosphazene (PPHOS) polymers that are colinked to hydroxyapatite materials to introduce a novel concept of injectable ceramic materials. PPHOS materials are designed out of a nitrogen and phosphate backbone and contain substituted amino acid side groups, which have been demonstrated to help the biocompatibility and mechanical properties of the polymers.[38] Initial studies on PPHOS have demonstrated these polymers to be ideal for cellular attachment, especially that of osteoblast cells, and the promotion of bone in in vivo rat and rabbit bone models.[39,40] In addition, histocompatibility studies have demonstrated these materials to be safe and ideal for tissue and bony ingrowth.[41] These injectable polymeric materials may become ideal delivery systems for BMP application. For instance, studies have demonstrated that the combination of PPHOS with hydroxyapatite creates an injectable paste that hardens at body temperature and produces significant bone formation in a tibial defect model. The delivery of a hybrid BMP-PPHOS matrix material could further potentiate the bone-inducing effects of BMP while simultaneously providing biomechanical integrity. These injectable materials along with other similar developments are promising alternatives that could play a future role in the augmentation of bone fusion, fracture treatment, and nonunion repair in tibia, foot, and ankle surgery.

Electrospinning has provided opportunities to develop materials that are appropriate for bone healing and BMP application. Human osteoblast cells cultured on electrospun polyester polymer scaffolds composed of varying concentration ratios of polylactic-co-glycolic acid (PLAGA) were observed to grow in significantly high numbers in the short and long term periods.[42] The same research group examined the efficacy of a BMP-7/PLAGA polymer matrix in inducing osteoblast expression and in vitro bone formation using rabbit muscle–derived stromal cells (**Fig. 1**). Their results confirmed that muscle-derived cells attached and proliferated on the PLAGA substrates and that BMP-7 released from PLAGA induced the muscle-derived cells to increase bone marker expression.[43] These results further demonstrate the

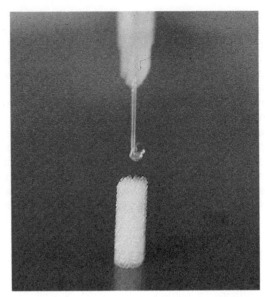

Fig. 1. rhOP-1 (BMP-7) being applied to 3-dimensional sintered PLAGA matrix (patent protected) for use as a bone graft substitute and delivery of the growth factor.

feasibility of the clinical application of BMP through combined BMP-polymer applications for bone tissue engineering.

The application of BMP for soft tissue repair has also been increasingly investigated in recent years. Growth/differentiation factor (GDF)-5, GDF-6, and GDF-7 (also known as BMP-14, BMP-13, and BMP-12, respectively) have been shown to be key factors in tendon repair.[44] GDF treatment induces cell proliferation, increases collagen

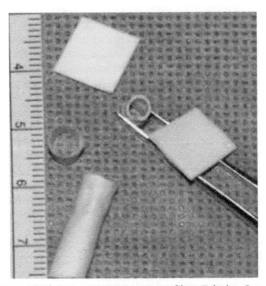

Fig. 2. Tissue Engineered Electrospun PLAGA Nanofiber Tubular Construct (patent protected). This construct has applications for the repair and regeneration of bone, soft tissue, and nerves, as well as the delivery of growth factors.

synthesis, and improves organization of the extracellular matrix. GDFs have also been shown to increase the transcription of multiple genes involved in tendon repair.[45] Park and colleagues[46] recently demonstrated that in vitro GDF-5 treatment can induce tendonogenic differentiation of adipose-derived mesenchymal cells from rats. A recent study showed that GDF-5 treatment after repair of Achilles tendon tenotomies led to improved collagen organization compared with controls in a murine model.[47] Animal studies evaluating the delivery of GDF-5 on electrospun polymer scaffolds for the regeneration of tendon defects are underway (**Fig. 2**). The combined use of GDF-5, stem cells, and polymer constructs may have a role in tendon repair of the foot and ankle in the future.

SUMMARY

The use of GDFs, especially BMPs, in foot and ankle surgery is evolving. Their application in fracture treatment, arthrodesis, and nonunion repair is becoming increasingly common. Current results and outcomes are promising, although more well-designed, large, multicenter clinical trials are needed. Tissue engineered innovations combining polymer, stem cell, and growth factor technologies may further advance the application of BMPs in bone, tendon, and soft tissue healing and repair in tibia, foot, and ankle surgery in the future.

REFERENCES

1. Woolverton CJ, Fulton JA, Lopina ST, et al. Mimicking the natural tissue environment. In: Lewandrowski K, Wise DL, Trantolo DJ, et al, editors. Tissue engineering and biodegradable equivalents: scientific and applications. New York: Marcel Dekkar; 2002. p. 43–75.
2. Pariente JL, Kim BS, Atala A. In vitro biocompatibility assessment of naturally derived and synthetic biomaterials using normal human urothelial cells. J Biomed Mater Res 2001;55(1):33–9.
3. Shum-Tim D, Stock U, Hrkach J, et al. Tissue engineering of autologous aorta using a new biodegradable polymer. Ann Thorac Surg 1999;68(6):2298–304 [discussion: 2305].
4. Margulis A, Zhang W, Garlick JA. In vitro fabrication of engineered human skin. Methods Mol Biol 2005;289:61–70.
5. Cao YL, Lach E, Kim TH, et al. Tissue-engineered nipple reconstruction. Plast Reconstr Surg 1998;102(7):2293–8.
6. Vandenburgh H, Del Tatto M, Shansky J, et al. Tissue-engineered skeletal muscle organoids for reversible gene therapy. Hum Gene Ther 1996;7(17):2195–200.
7. Frisbie DD, Lu Y, Kawcak CE, et al. In vivo evaluation of autologous cartilage fragment-loaded scaffolds implanted into equine articular defects and compared with autologous chondrocyte implantation. Am J Sports Med 2009;37(Suppl 1): 71S–80S.
8. Isogai N, Landis W, Kim TH, et al. Formation of phalanges and small joints by tissue-engineering. J Bone Joint Surg Am 1999;81(3):306–16.
9. Laurencin C, Khan Y, El-Amin SF. Bone graft substitutes. Expert Rev Med Devices 2006;3(1):49–57.
10. Khan Y, Yaszemski MJ, Mikos AG, et al. Tissue engineering of bone: material and matrix considerations. J Bone Joint Surg Am 2008;90(Suppl 1):36–42.
11. Taylor ED, Khan Y, Laurencin CT. Tissue engineering of bone: a primer for the practicing hand surgeon. J Hand Surg Am 2009;34(1):164–6.

12. Novicoff WM, Manaswi A, Hogan MV, et al. Critical analysis of the evidence for current technologies in bone-healing and repair. J Bone Joint Surg Am 2008; 90(Suppl 1):85–91.
13. Weinraub GM. Orthobiologics. Clin Podiatr Med Surg 2005;22(4):xiii–xxiv.
14. Schuberth JM, DiDomenico LA, Mendicino RW. The utility and effectiveness of bone morphogenetic protein in foot and ankle surgery. J Foot Ankle Surg 2009; 48(3):309–14.
15. Galois L, Mainard D, Pfeffer F, et al. Use of B-tricalcium phosphate in foot and ankle surgery: a report of 20 cases. Foot Ankle Surg 2001;7(4):217–27.
16. Laurencin CT, Khan Y, Kofron M, et al. The ABJS Nicolas Andry award: tissue engineering of bone and ligament: a 15-year perspective. Clin Orthop Relat Res 2006;447:221–36.
17. Urist MR. A morphogenetic matrix for differentiation of bone tissue. Calcif Tissue Res 1970;(Suppl):98–101.
18. Urist MR, Strates BS. Bone morphogenetic protein. J Dent Res 1971;50(6): 1392–406.
19. Assoian RK, Komoriya A, Meyers CA, et al. Transforming growth factor-beta in human platelets. Identification of a major storage site, purification, and characterization. J Biol Chem 1983;258(11):7155–60.
20. Abe E. Function of BMPs and BMP antagonists in adult bone. Ann N Y Acad Sci 2006;1068:41–53.
21. Guo X, Wang XF. Signaling cross-talk between TGF-beta/BMP and other pathways. Cell Res 2009;19(1):71–88.
22. Wu X, Shi W, Cao X. Multiplicity of BMP signaling in skeletal development. Ann N Y Acad Sci 2007;1116:29–49.
23. Valdes MA, Thakur NA, Namdari S, et al. Recombinant bone morphogenic protein-2 in orthopaedic surgery: a review. Arch Orthop Trauma Surg 2009; 129(12):1651–7.
24. Axelrad TW, Einhorn TA. Bone morphogenetic proteins in orthopaedic surgery. Cytokine Growth Factor Rev 2009;20(5–6):481–8.
25. Bibbo C, Haskell MD. Recombinant bone morphogenetic protein-2 (rhBMP-2) in high-risk foot and ankle surgery: surgical techniques and preliminary results of a prospective, intention-to-treat study. Tech Foot Ankle Surg 2007;6(2):71–9.
26. Bibbo C, Patel DV, Haskell MD. Recombinant bone morphogenetic protein-2 (rhBMP-2) in high-risk ankle and hindfoot fusions. Foot Ankle Int 2009;30(7): 597–603.
27. Kanakaris NK, Mallina R, Calori GM, et al. Use of bone morphogenetic proteins in arthrodesis: clinical results. Injury 2009;40(Suppl 3):S62–6.
28. McKee MD. Recombinant human bone morphogenic protein-7: applications for clinical trauma. J Orthop Trauma 2005;19(Suppl 10):S26–8.
29. Govender S, Csimma C, Genant HK, et al. Recombinant human bone morphogenetic protein-2 for treatment of open tibial fractures: a prospective, controlled, randomized study of four hundred and fifty patients. J Bone Joint Surg Am 2002;84(12):2123–34.
30. Swiontkowski MF, Aro HT, Donell S, et al. Recombinant human bone morphogenetic protein-2 in open tibial fractures. A subgroup analysis of data combined from two prospective randomized studies. J Bone Joint Surg Am 2006;88(6):1258–65.
31. Jones AL, Bucholz RW, Bosse MJ, et al. Recombinant human BMP-2 and allograft compared with autogenous bone graft for reconstruction of diaphyseal tibial fractures with cortical defects. A randomized, controlled trial. J Bone Joint Surg Am 2006;88(7):1431–41.

32. Ristiniemi J, Flinkkila T, Hyvonen P, et al. RhBMP-7 accelerates the healing in distal tibial fractures treated by external fixation. J Bone Joint Surg Br 2007; 89(2):265–72.

33. Zimmermann G, Wagner C, Schmeckenbecher K, et al. Treatment of tibial shaft non-unions: bone morphogenetic proteins versus autologous bone graft. Injury 2009;40(Suppl 3):S50–3.

34. Johnson EE, Urist MR, Finerman GA. Distal metaphyseal tibial nonunion. Deformity and bone loss treated by open reduction, internal fixation, and human bone morphogenetic protein (hBMP). Clin Orthop Relat Res 1990;250:234–40.

35. Friedlaender GE, Perry CR, Cole JD, et al. Osteogenic protein-1 (bone morphogenetic protein-7) in the treatment of tibial nonunions. J Bone Joint Surg Am 2001; 83(Suppl 1(Pt 2)):S151–8.

36. Moghaddam A, Elleser C, Biglari B, et al. Clinical application of BMP 7 in long bone non-unions. Arch Orthop Trauma Surg 2010;130(1):71–6.

37. Boraiah S, Paul O, Hawkes D, et al. Complications of recombinant human BMP-2 for treating complex tibial plateau fractures: a preliminary report. Clin Orthop Relat Res 2009;467(12):3257–62.

38. Sethuraman S, Nair LS, El-Amin S, et al. Mechanical properties and osteocompatibility of novel biodegradable alanine based polyphosphazenes: side group effects. Acta Biomater 2010;6(6):1931–7.

39. Passi P, Zadro A, Marsilio F, et al. Plain and drug loaded polyphosphazene membranes and microspheres in the treatment of rabbit bone defects. J Mater Sci Mater Med 2000;11(10):643–54.

40. Sethuraman S, Nair LS, El-Amin S, et al. In vivo biodegradability and biocompatibility evaluation of novel alanine ester based polyphosphazenes in a rat model. J Biomed Mater Res A 2006;77(4):679–87.

41. Sethuraman S, Nair LS, El-Amin S, et al. Development and characterization of biodegradable nanocomposite injectables for orthopaedic applications based on polyphosphazenes. J Biomater Sci Polym Ed 2010. [Epub ahead of print].

42. El-Amin SF, Botchwey E, Tuli R, et al. Human osteoblast cells: isolation, characterization, and growth on polymers for musculoskeletal tissue engineering. J Biomed Mater Res A 2006;76(3):439–49.

43. Lu HH, Kofron MD, El-Amin SF, et al. In vitro bone formation using muscle-derived cells: a new paradigm for bone tissue engineering using polymer-bone morphogenetic protein matrices. Biochem Biophys Res Commun 2003;305(4):882–9.

44. Wolfman NM, Hattersley G, Cox K, et al. Ectopic induction of tendon and ligament in rats by growth and differentiation factors 5, 6, and 7, members of the TGF-beta gene family. J Clin Invest 1997;100(2):321–30.

45. James R, Kesturu G, Balian G, et al. Tendon: biology, biomechanics, repair, growth factors, and evolving treatment options. J Hand Surg Am 2008;33(1):102–12.

46. Park A, Hogan MV, Kesturu GS, et al. Adipose-derived mesenchymal stem cells treated with growth differentiation factor-5 express tendon-specific markers. Tissue Eng Part A 2010;16(9):2941–51.

47. Hogan M, Girish K, James R, et al. Growth differentiation factor-5 regulation of extracellular matrix gene expression in murine tendon fibroblasts. J Tissue Eng Regen Med 2010. [Epub ahead of print].

The Use of Proximal and Distal Tibial Bone Graft in Foot and Ankle Procedures

Ian G. Winson, MBChB, FRCS*, Andrew Higgs, MBBS, FRACS

KEYWORDS

- Iliac crest • Proximal tibia • Distal tibia • Bone graft
- Foot and ankle surgery

Autologous bone grafting techniques are regularly used in foot and ankle surgery. The use of autologous bone has theoretical advantages over the use of allograft and other bone substitutes because of its superior integration and also because it negates the potential risk of immunologic and infectious complications associated with the use of allograft. Further advantages of autologous bone are that it has all the characteristics of a potent osteoinductive, osteoconductive, and osteogenic material.[1]

Traditionally, autologous bone is harvested from the anterior iliac crest. The anterior iliac crest is easily accessible and can provide large quantities of cancellous and cortical bone. The ability to obtain tricortical grafts makes the iliac crest ideal in situations in which structural support may be required. It is argued that the iliac crest may offer an advantage with regard to greater osteogenic potential as a result of high marrow content. Histologic studies show that the bone from the iliac crest differs from the tibial bone, with the presence of more active hematopoietic marrow and a greater osteogenic surface.[2] The iliac crest graft contains more hematopoietic marrow, whereas the tibial graft medullary spaces largely contain fat.[2] Therefore, from a cellular point of view it may seem justified to use iliac crest graft, given the presence of hematopoietic material and its potential contribution to osteogenesis. Counter to this argument is the finding that the contribution to bone formation from hematopoietic cells is minimal.[3] On balance, the anterior iliac crest can be regarded as the gold standard site for bone graft harvest. Despite this finding, many clinicians recognize considerable disadvantages to using this site for graft harvest during foot and ankle surgery. The most obvious problem is related to its anatomic location, requiring the preparation of a second surgical site. It has been

Avon Orthopaedic Centre, Southmead Hospital, Bristol BS10 5NB, UK
* Corresponding author. Spire Hospital Bristol, Sports and Orthopaedics Clinic, Redland Hill, Durdham Down, Bristol, BS6 6UT, UK
E-mail address: ianwinson@doctors.org.uk

Foot Ankle Clin N Am 15 (2010) 553–558
doi:10.1016/j.fcl.2010.07.005
1083-7515/10/$ – see front matter © 2010 Elsevier Inc. All rights reserved.

argued that the second surgical site is advantageous and enables the assistant to harvest the graft simultaneously and so save time. Good results using unicortical anterior iliac crest graft are reported with a self-reported satisfaction rate of 90%.[4] The same studies also report an incidence of residual pain in 10% of patients and residual numbness surrounding the harvest site in 9%. The investigators regard these complications as minor and report the overall incidence of minor complications as 9.5%. The authors do not support that iliac crest bone graft saves time. A second assistant can just as easily obtain graft from the proximal tibia at the same time as the index procedure.

Many studies have highlighted a higher potential for complications with the use of the anterior iliac crest. These complications can be judged as minor or major, and the overall complication rate from anterior iliac crest bone graft has been reported to be a high as 43%.[2] The most common complications are nerve injury, hematoma, and postoperative pain.[5,6] During foot and ankle surgery, it is often not necessary to obtain large quantities of bone graft. In the authors' experience, most foot and ankle cases that require bone graft need only small quantities of the graft, with a maximum of 30 cc. The literature suggests that the amount of graft material required in foot and ankle surgery is generally small. Rosenfeld and colleagues[7] in their study support this opinion. The investigators show comparable union rates of 96% during triple arthrodesis without the use of any supplementary bone graft, other than that available locally. The authors agree with this experience and only use distant autologous graft on the rare occasion in which there is a specific problem with using more local sites.

Intuitively, it also makes sense that the bone graft donor site in close proximity to that of the primary surgical site is used. This use can simplify surgical preparation and potentially minimizes the morbidity associated with autologous graft harvest, which could impair rehabilitation and postoperative recovery. It is well reported that early postoperative pain, associated with iliac crest grafting, can hinder mobility. Pain from the iliac crest graft site is greater in 27% of cases than that from the index foot and ankle procedure.[4]

These reasons make both the proximal and distal tibial donor sites attractive options during foot and ankle surgery. Well-reported literature to date supports the use of these sites in foot and ankle surgery because of the low associated complication rates from using these sites.

To date, there are no prospective randomized controlled trials that compare the use of different graft donor sites during foot and ankle surgery. A review of the current literature suggests that the proximal and distal tibial donor sites offer a distinct advantage over the iliac crest during foot and ankle surgery by reducing the complication rate with no discernible loss of efficacy.

PROXIMAL TIBIA

The proximal tibia has obvious advantages because of its anatomic location. Graft can be obtained from the ipsilateral limb and distal to the tourniquet, without change in patient position. It is also included easily within the same operative field. Graft can be taken from both the medial and the lateral aspect of the proximal tibia, and exposure is often more easily obtained because of the smaller quantity of subcutaneous fat present in the proximal tibia than in the iliac crest. Significant amounts of graft can be obtained from this site, and an estimate of 30 cc is not uncommonly reported.[8] According to a study by Ahlmann and colleagues,[5] this amount compares reasonably with the 55 cc that is harvested on average from the anterior iliac crest, thus highlighting the significant quantity that can be obtained from this site. In the authors' clinical practice, the proximal tibia provides quantities of grafts, which are more than adequate for most of the surgeries involving the foot and ankle.

Whitehouse and colleagues[9] performed a retrospective review of 148 procedures of foot and ankle arthrodesis using bone graft from the proximal tibia, which was performed over a period of 5 years, with a minimum follow-up of 3 months.[9] No major complications occurred during the study period. Most patients had either no pain (78%) or very mild pain (20%) at the graft harvest site immediately after surgery. At follow-up, 96% of patients had no pain and only 4% had mild pain, while 2.7% had a minor sensory disturbance of less than 1 cm^2. No difficulty in obtaining sufficient graft from the proximal tibia was experienced during the surgery. The postoperative weight-bearing status or rehabilitative protocol was not altered by the grafting procedure, and no fractures occurred during the study period. The authors conclude that the proximal tibia is a reliable and safe site of bone harvest in patients undergoing elective foot and ankle surgery.

O'Keeffe and colleagues[10] retrospectively reviewed 230 cases of bone grafting associated with lower extremity fractures and nonunions. Although the study was not isolated to surgery performed on the foot and ankle, only a 1.3% complication rate was reported. One tibial eminence fracture, one hematoma, and one case of superficial wound infection were reported. No reports of sensory loss or altered sensation occurred around the region of the harvest site.

Alt and colleagues[11] reported on a series of 54 cases during their retrospective review of the use of proximal tibial bone graft. This study was not isolated to grafting of the foot and ankle and also included other sites. All patients were permitted to weight bear as tolerated through the donor limb, and no subsequent fractures were reported. No major complications occurred, although a minor complication of hematoma, but no other complication, was observed in 1.9% of the patients.

The study by Geideman and colleagues[8] reported the success of the proximal tibia as a donor site. The review included a cohort of 155 patients undergoing elective foot and ankle reconstruction. Postoperative weight-bearing status was decided on according to the primary procedure. No major complications, in particular fractures, were reported during the study period. Minor complications were nonetheless reported; 3 cases of temporary nerve injury and 1 hematoma, resulting in an incidence of 2.6% for minor complications. Surprisingly, all these articles show consistent low complication rates.

Authors' Preferred Technique for Proximal Tibial Autologous Graft Harvest

The lower limb is prepped and draped, so to include the proximal tibial metaphysis within the operative field. An above-knee tourniquet, although not essential, is preferred, if not contraindicated. A 3-cm longitudinal incision measuring a thumb's breadth is then made medially and just tending distally to the tibial tuberosity.

Care is taken to avoid and preserve the inferior patella and saphenous nerve. Using a periosteal elevator, the underlying proximal tibia is exposed. Using a 2.7-mm drill, 4 drill holes are placed through the cortex to form a square of 1 × 1 cm^2 (**Fig. 1**).

Thus, the circular corners produced by the drill distribute the stress more evenly at the corners of the window. A 1-cm osteotome is then used to join these holes and gain access to the proximal tibia. Standard curettes can be used to collect the graft, supplemented by curved artery forceps. At the end of the procedure, the window is replaced and the wound closed in a standard fashion without drainage. The postoperative weight-bearing status is dictated by the primary procedure.

Editor's note: Some controversy still remains over the merits of backfilling the proximal tibial bone graft site. The authors do not routinely fill the donor site and have had

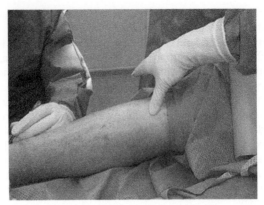

Fig. 1. A thumb-distance incision medial to the tibial tuberosity.

no negative outcomes from this practice. At my hospital, Dr Robert Brumback harvests a sometimes very large amount of cancellous bone from the proximal tibia (for long bone defects) and backfills the graft site with allograft bone chips; I do the same. For smaller harvest amounts, many surgeons chose not to back fill, like Dr Gregory Guyton prefers. I caution against backfilling with Pro-Osteon (coralline calcium phosphate) because the later radiographic appearance of the slowly resorbing material can mimic a tumor and cause undue concern.

DISTAL TIBIA

The distal tibia also offers opportunistic access to small but sometimes sufficient quantities of autologous cancellous autograft during foot and ankle surgery. The distal tibia can be approached from either medial or lateral aspects and the graft obtained. As when harvesting cancellous bone from the proximal tibia, certain principles apply. Preferably, circular windows should be fashioned because these reduce the effect of the stress riser that occurs at acute angles. Perhaps more relevant to the distal tibia is that the graft should be taken distal to the metaphyseal-diaphyseal junction because fractures can occur. The geometric configuration of the distal tibia should be borne in mind when attempting to harvest graft from this site, and every effort should be made to ensure that only the metaphyseal portion of the bone is violated. For this reason, the authors regard the upper tibial site as being preferable.

Evidence can also be found within the literature to support the upper tibial site. Because of the occasional report of major complications, in particular fracture, this evidence is not as compelling or as comprehensive as that supporting the use of the proximal tibia.

In a study by Raikin and colleagues,[12] 70 patients undergoing foot and ankle arthrodesis surgery with graft taken from the distal tibia were reported to have no major complications and only 7% minor complications. These minor complications were all caused by irritation of the saphenous nerve. The investigators also reported that all patients were satisfied with the procedure and would choose to undergo the procedure again.

Danziger and colleagues,[13] in a study of 40 patients, reported exceptionally positive results at an average follow-up of 23.3 months. No complications related to the distal tibial donor site were reported.

A further study by Weiss and colleagues[14] also showed positive results. In a prospective study, with a minimum follow-up of 6 months, excellent results in 28 feet were reported. The investigators used a medial incision and were able to obtain an average of 2.6 cc of graft. No major complications were reported. Minor complications included 2 superficial wound infections, 3 cases of skin irritation, and 1 nonunion. The investigators summarized their experience as being positive; however, the study does echo some concerns over the quantity of available graft. However, the small quantity is rarely an issue when the grafting requires only a small amount of graft in the foot and ankle.

Chou and colleagues,[15] in their review of 100 cases, reported that stress fractures occur. The investigators reported the occurrence of 4 stress fractures related to the donor site. All fractures were successfully treated by immobilization.

The occurrence of stress fractures has also been encountered at the authors' institution, with 2 fractures related to the distal graft site. This problem has never been seen in proximal graft sites.

Authors' Preferred Technique for Distal Tibial Autologous Graft Harvest

The distal tibia should be approached from the medial side, posterior to the saphenous nerve and vein. Care should be taken to avoid entering the ankle joint or straying proximally into the distal tibial diaphysis. Blunt dissection is performed, and the bone is exposed subperiosteally. As in the proximal tibia, graft can be obtained through an oval cortical window on this occasion. A 2.7-mm drill bit is used to fashion 4 holes into an oval template. An osteotome is used to complete the corticotomy, and the window is flipped outward. Graft is then collected with a curette, and then the window and soft tissues are closed. It is generally accepted that with this technique, less amounts of graft are obtained and that the rate of major complications, such as fracture, is greater. If care is taken with smaller graft requirements, the graft is easily obtained.

SUMMARY

Bone graft that may be required during foot and ankle surgery rarely requires quantities to warrant the iliac crest as the primary choice for grafting. Despite its superior histologic appearance, there is no evidence to support that this graft site offers any potential advantage to achieving greater union rates in surgery isolated to the foot and ankle. Given that the obtaining of graft from the iliac crest is also associated with a generally higher complication rate, the authors support and recommend the use of alternative sites, particularly the proximal tibia, as the first site of choice for the acquirement of autologous bone during foot and ankle surgery.

REFERENCES

1. Finkemeier CG. Bone-grafting and bone-graft substitutes. J Bone Joint Surg Am 2002;84:454–64.
2. Hahne J, Chiodo CP, Wilson MG. Autogenous bone grafts in foot and ankle surgery. The Orthopaedic Journal at Harvard Medical School 2007;9:113–6 [online].
3. Gray JC, Elves MW. Early osteogenesis in compact bone isograft: a quantitative study of contributions of the different graft cells. Calcif Tissue Int 1979;29:225–37.
4. DeOrio JK, Farber DC. Morbidity associated with anterior iliac crest bone grafting in foot and ankle surgery. Foot Ankle Int 2005;26:147–51.

5. Ahlmann E, Patzakis M, Roidis N, et al. Comparison of anterior and posterioriliac crest bone grafts in terms of harvest-site morbidity and functional outcomes. J Bone Joint Surg Am 2002;84:716–20.
6. Arrington ED, Smith WJ, Chambers HG, et al. Complications of iliac crest bone harvesting. Clin Orthop Relat Res 1996;329:300–9.
7. Rosenfeld PF, Budgen SA, Saxby TS. Triple arthrodesis: is bone grafting necessary? J Bone Joint Surg Br 2005;87:175–8.
8. Geideman W, Early JS, Brodsky J. Clinical results of harvesting autogenous cancellous graft from the ipsilateral proximal tibia for use in foot and ankle surgery. Foot Ankle Int 2004;25:451–5.
9. Whitehouse MR, Lankester BJA, Winson IG, et al. Bone graft harvest from the proximal tibia in foot and ankle arthodesis surgery. Foot Ankle Int 2006;27(11): 913–6.
10. O'Keeffe RM, Riemer BL, Butterfield SL. Harvesting of autogenous cancellous bone graft from the proximal tibial metaphysis. A review of 230 cases. J Orthop Trauma 1991;5:469–74.
11. Alt V, Nawab A, Seligson D. Bone grafting from the proximal tibia. J Trauma 1999; 47(3):555–7 five.
12. Raikin SM, Brislin K. Local bone graft harvested from the distal tibia or calcaneus for surgery of the foot and ankle. Foot Ankle Int 2005;26:449–53.
13. Danziger MB, Abdo RV, Decker JE. Distal tibial bone graft for arthrodessis of the foot and ankle. Foot Ankle Int 1995;16:187–90.
14. Weiss GA, Saxby T. Distal tibial bone graft for foot and ankle surgery. Foot Ankle Surg 1998;4:93–7.
15. Chou LB, Mann RA, Coughlin MJ, et al. Stress fracture as a complication of autogenous bone graft harvest from the distal tibia. Foot Ankle Int 2007;28: 199–201.

Synthetic Bone Grafting in Foot and Ankle Surgery

Vinod K. Panchbhavi, MD, FRCS (Eng)

KEYWORDS

• Calcium sulfate • Calcium phosphate • Synthetic bone graft

SYNTHETIC BONE GRAFTS

Bone grafts are used by surgeons in the management of a wide variety of conditions, including tumors, trauma, and infection.[1] Autografts have long been held as the gold standard for bone graft procedures because they contain osteogenic bone cells, marrow cells, and an osteoconductive collagen matrix suitable for new and existing bone-cell attachment and migration as well as osteoinductive proteins and factors endogenous to bone.[2] In addition, autogenous bone is not antigenic but the harvesting of autogenous bone requires a second operation and can be associated with substantial donor site morbidity and complications. The common problems that have been reported include pain at the donor site, meralgia paraesthetica as a result of injury to the lateral femoral cutaneous nerve, injury of the superior gluteal artery, pelvic fracture, hematoma, infection, and gait disturbances.[3–6] Furthermore, the amount of autogenous bone available for harvesting is limited and may be insufficient to fill large osseous defects. The quality of the harvested autogenous bone is also variable.

One alternative to autograft is allograft, or tissue taken from a cadaver. With allografts limited supply is less of a problem but there is a potential for disease transmission from donor to recipient.[7] Additional allograft complications have been reported at the 10-year mark, with as many as 30% to 60% of allograft implants encountering some sort of complication that may lead to failure of the structural allograft.[8–10] Given the shortcomings of autografts and allografts and the growing demand for bone grafts, several alternative synthetic materials are being investigated. They share numerous advantages over autografts and allografts, including their unlimited supply, easy sterilization, and easy storage.

The synthetic bone graft substitutes described later are mainly used for their osteoconductive abilities. The term osteoconduction refers to a process in which

The author has nothing to disclose.

Division of Foot & Ankle Surgery, Department of Orthopedic Surgery, University of Texas Medical Branch, 301, University Boulevard, Galveston, TX 77555-0165, USA

E-mail address: vkpanchb@utmb.edu

doi:10.1016/j.fcl.2010.07.004
1083-7515/10/$ – see front matter © 2010 Elsevier Inc. All rights reserved.

foot.theclinics.com

the three-dimensional structure of a substance is conducive for the ongrowth and/or ingrowth of newly formed bone. Osteoconductive materials essentially provide a substrate, or matrix, that supports the migration, attachment, and proliferation of mesenchymal stem cells, which then differentiate into osteoprogenitor cells that form bone. These substances typically have a microscopic structure similar to that of cancellous bone as well as attractive surface kinetics. During osteoconductive bone ingrowth, capillaries, perivascular tissue, and osteoprogenitor cells migrate into the bone graft substitute; newly formed bone is produced within its porous spaces.[11,12] Pore size and porosity are important characteristics of bone graft substitutes. No osseous ingrowth occurs with pore sizes of 15 to 40 μm. Osteoid formation requires minimum pore sizes of 100 μm; pore sizes of 150 to 500 μm are reported to be ideal for osseous ingrowth.[13] However, some investigators have reported that pore size may be less critical than the presence of interconnecting pores for osseous ingrowth. Interconnecting pores prevent the formation of blind alleys, which are associated with low oxygen tension; low oxygen tension prevents osteoprogenitor cells from differentiating into osteoblasts.[14]

In addition to providing a mechanical buttress, these osteoconductive scaffolds may prevent soft tissue from occluding the space and hindering bone formation. Peltier and Jones[15] showed that osteoconduction requires the bone graft substitute to have a resorption rate similar to the rate of new bone formation. If the rate of resorption is faster than the rate of bone growth, the new bone does not have a scaffold on which to travel. Conversely, if the graft material resorbs too slowly, it may stay in the osseous defect and block the ingrowth of new bone.

Ceramics used as scaffolds for fracture repair can be subdivided into 3 main categories by their chemical reactivity following transplant: bioabsorbable ceramics, bioactive ceramics, and bioinert ceramics.[16] Bioabsorbable and bioactive substances are able to physically bond directly to the host bed, whereas bioinert ones never actually bond to the bone. Nonbiodegradable polymers form another class of osteoconductive grafts.[17]

Bioabsorbable ceramics were the first synthetic materials used in bone transplantation. The ones that are commonly used include calcium sulfate, calcium phosphate, and tricalcium phosphate (TCP). These products vary considerably in their chemical composition, structural strength, and resorption/remodeling rates.[18] They may be used selectively or in combination. The surgeon must understand the chemical composition, physical characteristics, and bioactivity of various synthetic substitutes and the differences between them to select a bone graft substitute that provides the properties desired for a specific clinical situation.

Although bone graft substitutes are subject to varying degrees of regulatory scrutiny, specific proof of efficacy is not always required.[19] Most bone graft substitutes currently marketed in the United States have been approved through a less stringent premarket notification (510[k]). In this process, the manufacturer must provide data showing that the new product is substantially equivalent to an already approved legally marketed device, which includes products commercially distributed before the May 28, 1976, Medical Device Amendment.[19] Marketing claims are not always well supported by published data.[20]

There are a limited number of clinical studies and a lack of direct comparison studies between these products. In addition, the difficulty in showing new bone formation varies by anatomic region. Therefore, validation of the effectiveness of a bone graft substitute in one anatomic location may not be predictive of its performance in another. Thus, surgeons should avoid extrapolating available clinical evidence to other anatomic areas.

This article is a review of the chemical, physical, and biologic characteristics of synthetic bone graft substitutes used in foot and ankle surgery and of the available experimental and clinical studies.

Calcium Sulfate

Calcium sulfate in the form of a hemihydrate is more commonly known to orthopedic surgeons as plaster of Paris, a material used for splinting and casting. When the hemihydrate form of calcium sulfate ($CaSO_4 \cdot 0.5H_2O$) is mixed with water, a dihydrate known as gypsum ($CaSO_4 \cdot 2H_2O$) is formed. The hemihydrate form of calcium sulfate (CaO_4S), a bioabsorbable ceramic, is prepared by heating gypsum.

Calcium sulfate is one of the oldest bone graft substitutes. Its reported use dates to 1892. Calcium sulfate was first used by Dreesmann[21] to obliterate bone cavities caused by tuberculosis. Peltier[22] became the first American to report on the use of calcium sulfate as a bone graft substitute. He established that calcium sulfate can be resorbed and replaced by bone in vivo. Peltier[23] further concluded that the presence of calcium sulfate in a wound did not inhibit the formation of bone and that it was removed from the site of implantation irrespective of whether new bone formation occurred. Infection in wounds containing calcium sulfate was not complicated by sequestration of the material; it either drained out or was absorbed. Peltier and Jones[15] found that calcium sulfate is safe to use in a variety of cavitary bone defects, that it is completely resorbed, and that regeneration of bone occurred in weeks to months. However, despite its initial success, the use of calcium sulfate was later associated with inconsistent results. This situation may have been due to impurities and a nonuniform structure of the calcium sulfate crystals. Subsequent improvements in the production of calcium sulfate have resulted in a high-grade material that is more suitable for surgical applications. Contemporary medical-grade calcium sulfate is inexpensive, can be sterilized and prepared easily, has an indefinite shelf life, and can be used in various sizes of osseous defects. Its resorption can also be monitored radiographically because it is radiopaque.[24,25]

Calcium sulfate works in an osteoconductive manner, providing a scaffold into which new bone can grow. Walsh and colleagues[26] hypothesized that the mechanism of bone regenerative action of calcium sulfate is related to the local acidity produced during its resorption. These investigators postulated that in a confined cancellous defect, this local acidity results in demineralization of the adjacent bone, with a release of matrix-bound bone morphogenetic proteins that have a stimulatory effect on bone formation. It has been shown that osteoblasts attach to calcium salts.

In cultures of rat bone, Sidqui and colleagues[27] observed that osteoblasts attach to the surface of calcium sulfate pellets, and osteoclasts can resorb the mineral in vitro. A similar mechanism in vivo may be responsible for the resorption and rapid regeneration of bone defects by calcium sulfate.[28] During the process of resorption, there is vascular infiltration, osteoid deposition, and ultimately restoration of the defect with new mineralized bone trabeculae. The new bone is seen layering on the microscopic residual of $CaSO_4$ as it is substantially resorbed in the 6-week period.[26,29,30]

In a canine humeral model, Turner and colleagues[31] studied bone regeneration around pellets of calcium sulfate. Six weeks after implantation, thin trabeculae of new bone spanned the space between pellets, and by 24 weeks the pellets had resorbed and the bone regeneration was qualitatively similar to that seen after autogenous bone grafting indistinguishable by volume or by histologic features from that of autograft-filled defects. New trabeculae of bone are easily distinguishable on radiographs from the amorphous calcium sulfate pellets.

As with other calcium-based bone graft substitutes, $CaSO_4$ is well tolerated, evoking minimal inflammatory or foreign body reaction.[19,29-31] The rapid 6-week resorption period seems ideal for early bone repair.[29-31] However, the rapid resorption may be responsible for the development in some clinical applications of serous drainage, which usually resolves spontaneously.[32] It has been theorized that this serous drainage is the result of the osmotic effect of the calcium sulfate and that it subsides with calcium sulfate resorption.[33]

Calcium sulfate is available either as individual pellets or as a powder that can be mixed in solution to form an injectable paste or molded to form desired shapes. Its compressive strength is similar to that of cancellous bone.[34] Some setting solutions for use with the powder are proprietary, and these solutions may differ between companies.[33]

Calcium sulfate is available in a variety of forms, the most common being hard pellets of calcium sulfate hydrate (eg, Osteoset, Wright Medical Technology, Arlington, TN, USA; JAX, Smith & Nephew, Memphis, TN, USA; Calceon, Synthes, Paoli, PA, USA). Calcium sulfate hemihydrate is a powder that hardens when mixed with a diluent. Minimally invasive injectable graft (MIIG, Wright Medical) is an injectable calcium sulfate that hardens in vivo, allowing for filling voids percutaneously. Boneplast bone void filler (Interpore Cross International, Irvine, CA) and Osteoset T (Wright Medical) can be fashioned into beads and impregnated with antibiotics for local antibiotic treatment, thereby providing a major advantage in the treatment of infected bone.

Use of calcium sulfate alone or in combination to fill bone defects has been reported in several studies. Watson[35] reported promising results on the use of injectable calcium sulfate in 5 patients who sustained tibial plateau fracture and in 3 patients with tibial pilon fracture. Borelli and colleagues[36] used a mixture of autogenous iliac crest bone graft and calcium sulfate to treat 19 patients with long-bone nonunions and 7 with acute fractures with large osseous defects. Calcium sulfate was used as a bone graft expander in conjunction with internal fixation. Union was successful following initial surgical treatment in 85% of patients. When autogenous bone graft is being placed to restore absent cortical bone, calcium sulfate may be used to fill the deeper intramedullary area; the bone graft is placed on top so that it remains in contact with the surrounding muscular soft-tissue bed.[33]

Gitelis and colleagues[37] reported healing in 21 of 23 patients with bony defects treated with calcium sulfate, either alone or in combination with demineralized bone matrix. Mirzayan and colleagues[25] described healing in 13 of 13 patients in their series with defects that resulted from treatment of benign bone tumors or osteomyelitis. All of the defects healed in a centripetal fashion, in which the more peripherally placed calcium sulfate pellets were resorbed first and the more central pellets were the last to disappear. The average time to healing was 13.4 weeks (range, 5–24 weeks). The rate of healing depended on the size of the lesion. In one patient, some calcification developed in the adjacent soft tissues because some of the calcium sulfate pellets had spilled out of the cavity intraoperatively. This calcification was seen to have disappeared on a 6-month follow-up radiograph. Kelly and colleagues[32] in a multicenter trial reported on use of calcium sulfate pellets alone or in combination with demineralized bone matrix, autograft, or bone marrow aspirate in 109 patients with bone defects caused by tumor (42%), trauma (36%), and other causes (22%), such as periprosthetic bone loss and fusion augmentation. These investigators found that patients who were treated with calcium sulfate pellets alone had a greater amount of bone ingrowth than those who were treated with a mixture of calcium sulfate pellets and other substances. Four patients developed serous wound drainage that was believed to be related to the calcium sulfate product.

Fracture stabilization in osteoporotic bones presents a special challenge. A variety of techniques are used to prevent failure of fixation and to improve purchase of implants. Injectable calcium sulfate has been used to augment purchase of the tibia pro fibular screws in internal fixation of an osteoporotic ankle fracture (**Figs. 1–5**).[38]

Calcium sulfate combined with antibiotics eliminates the dead space with gradual local release of antibiotics and has been used with good results in management of osteomyelitis, although this represents an off-label use of the product in the United States. McKee and colleagues[39] studied 24 patients with infected nonunions and bone defects treated with a $CaSO_4$ delivery system for local antibiotics. Infection was eradicated in 23 of the 24 patients and union was achieved in 10 of 16 nonunions. Postoperative draining sinuses present at the time of pellet resorption cleared spontaneously. It seems that the slow resorption of the $CaSO_4$ pellets and elution of the antibiotics maintained a prolonged delivery of local antibiotics. The calcium sulfate also may have permitted or facilitated new bone formation within the infected defects.

Calcium Phosphate

Calcium phosphate is available in a variety of forms and products, including ceramics, powders, and cements.[40] The various forms of calcium phosphate cement have

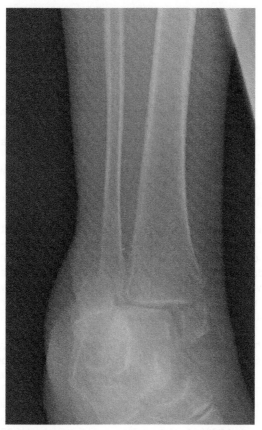

Fig. 1. Preoperative radiograph of an osteoporotic ankle fracture. (*Reproduced from* Panchbhavi VK. Augmentation of internal fixation of osteoporotic ankle fracture using injectable bone substitute. Tech Foot Ankle Surg 2007;6:265; with permission.)

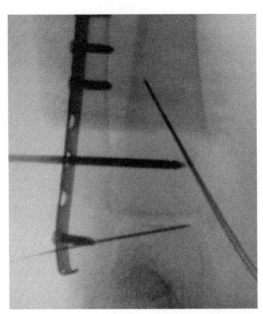

Fig. 2. Intraoperative fluoroscopy image showing the cannula in the screw hole. (*Reproduced from* Panchbhavi VK. Augmentation of internal fixation of osteoporotic ankle fracture using injectable bone substitute. Tech Foot Ankle Surg 2007;6:266; with permission.)

different mechanical and biologic resorption characteristics.[41] The injectable paste of inorganic calcium and phosphate hardens in situ and cures by a crystallization reaction in a nonexothermic reaction to form dahllite, a carbonated apatite similar to that found in the mineral phase of bone. The injectable nature of calcium phosphate cement was designed to facilitate percutaneous administration.[33,42] On implantation, the cements sets and begins to harden, and the cement interdigitates with the adjacent bone, thus forming a solid structure that is more mechanically stable than either cancellous bone graft or hydroxyapatite granules. It is bioabsorbable and compatible in vivo.[42]

Compared with cancellous bone grafts and other bone graft substitutes, calcium phosphate, when hardened, has a higher compressive strength (4–10 times greater than cancellous bone) and may be useful in preventing subsequent displacement or depression of reduced articular fragments. In materials testing, calcium phosphate cement has showed excellent strength in compression and strength equivalent to cancellous bone in tension (2 MPa).[43] But calcium phosphate cements do not provide a high level of structural support because they are brittle and have little tensile strength.[44,45]

Calcium phosphate first became available in the United States as Norian skeletal repair system (SRS) (Synthes, Paoli, PA, USA). It is now available from multiple manufacturers. Animal studies have shown that the material is gradually remodeled in a manner that is qualitatively similar to normal bone remodeling. Over time, calcium phosphate undergoes osteoclastic resorption, followed by the invasion of small blood vessels that become surrounded by circumferential lamellae of new bone.[42] Animal studies have shown that 95% of calcium phosphate is resorbed in 26 to 86 weeks.[46,47] Incomplete resorption after 6 months has been reported in animal studies,[41] and in 3 of 4 patients there was no change in the radiographic or computed tomography

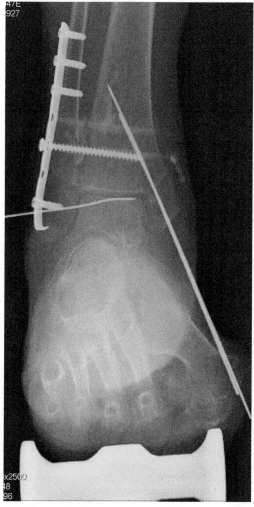

Fig. 3. Intraoperative radiograph showing calcium sulfate in the track along the screw holes. (*Reproduced from* Panchbhavi VK. Augmentation of internal fixation of osteoporotic ankle fracture using injectable bone substitute. Tech Foot Ankle Surg 2007;6:266; with permission.)

appearance of the cement at 18 months after the operation.[48] In humans, the histology of retrieved femoral heads previously implanted with Norian SRS showed remodeling processes identical to those observed in animal studies.[49]

Unlike calcium sulfate, which is crystalline, independent of the rate of resorption, and a true salt that can dissolve into Ca^{2+} and SO_4^{2-} ions, calcium phosphate materials, although crystalline, are dependent on the rate of resorption and are true ceramics and therefore do not dissolve within the joint. As a result, they may cause cartilage wear if left exposed in the intracapsular space.[50] Concerns therefore have been expressed about potential intraarticular extrusion of calcium phosphate when used in intraarticular fractures; however, no adverse sequelae have been reported when extrusion has occurred.[51] There do not seem to be any early adverse

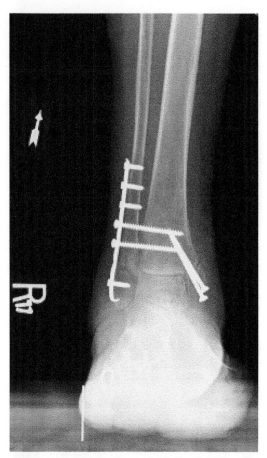

Fig. 4. Follow-up mortise view radiograph at 12 weeks showing no evidence of implant failure or displacement and complete resorbtion of calcium sulfate. (*Reproduced from* Panchbhavi VK. Augmentation of internal fixation of osteoporotic ankle fracture using injectable bone substitute. Tech Foot Ankle Surg 2007;6:267; with permission.)

effects, such as inflammation, and foreign body responses, to these ceramics when they are in a structural block arrangement.[51] However, small granules of material have been shown to elicit a foreign body giant cell reaction.[52,53]

Injectable calcium phosphate cements have been proposed as a tool to fill voids in metaphyseal bone, thereby improving host bone strength and the purchase of metal devices.[49] The most commonly used are the Norian SRS cement (Norian Corp, Cupertino, CA, USA) and the Bone Source (Stryker Howmedica Osteonics, Rutherford, NJ, USA). These cements are available as 2 components, one in powder form and the other as liquid, which are mixed manually or with a mixing machine in the operating room. After mixing, they are similar to toothpaste in appearance and can be easily injected in the area of interest.

A recent meta-analysis of 14 randomized, controlled trials, one of which involved calcaneal fractures, suggested that the use of calcium phosphate bone cement for the treatment of fractures is associated with the benefits of (1) less pain at the fracture

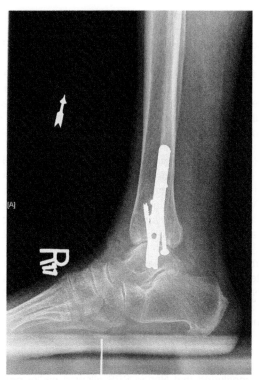

Fig. 5. Follow-up lateral view radiograph at 12 weeks showing no evidence of implant failure or displacement and complete resorbtion of calcium sulfate. (*Reproduced from* Panchbhavi VK. Augmentation of internal fixation of osteoporotic ankle fracture using injectable bone substitute. Tech Foot Ankle Surg 2007;6:267; with permission.)

site compared with that in controls managed with no bone graft or no bone graft substitutes and (2) a reduced risk for losing fracture reduction when compared with autogenous bone graft. The results of individual studies suggested improved functional outcomes in association with the use of calcium phosphate cement. This finding could be explained by the fact that patients in the calcium phosphate group had less pain and less risk for loss of reduction.[54]

Displaced intraarticular calcaneal fractures continue to be a therapeutic challenge for orthopedic surgeons. The goal of operative treatment is to restore the complex foot and ankle biomechanics by performing an anatomic reduction of the subtalar posterior facet and restoring calcaneal height and length.[55,56] The difficulty often arises in maintaining this reduction postoperatively. In axial loading injuries that cause displaced intraarticular calcaneal fractures, the trabecular cancellous bone of the calcaneus is crushed. Operative reduction leaves a sizable bone void beneath the elevated posterior facet. Despite stable internal fixation, evidence indicates that the presence of a bone void predisposes the calcaneus to collapse, resulting in a loss of both posterior facet reduction and calcaneal height.[57] Cancellous bone graft has not been shown to prevent collapse, and the biomechanical properties of polymethylmethacrylate (PMMA) make it an unattractive option.[57,58]

Thordarson and colleagues[59] performed a cadaver study that showed improved compressive strength and stability of the fixation of experimentally created calcaneal fractures when the construct was augmented with Norian SRS1. These investigators compared intraarticular calcaneal fractures fixed with standard internal fixation with those in which the osseous defect was filled with bone graft or SRS. In the specimens treated with the combination of hardware and SRS cement, cyclic loading produced significantly less deformation.

Schildhauer and colleagues[60] reported a series of 36 joint depression-type calcaneal fractures that had been treated with internal fixation augmented by calcium phosphate cement. They found that patients who had been allowed to bear weight as early as 3 weeks after the surgery had no radiographic evidence of loss of reduction, and there was no significant difference in functional outcome scores between patients who had been allowed to begin bearing weight before 6 weeks and those who began it after 6 weeks. However, the investigators did note an 11% infection rate. Seventy-five percent of the infections developed in smokers, and histologic evaluation of tissue from those patients showed no giant cells or eosinophils to suggest a foreign body or allergic reaction. Although this infection rate is an important outcome to consider, the investigators concluded that cement augmentation of internal fixation of joint depression-type calcaneal fractures allowed earlier weight bearing with no change in postoperative outcomes.

Recently, 2 European clinical studies have investigated the use of bioresorbable calcium phosphate paste (Biobon, the European equivalent of α-BSM (bone substitute material; Etex Corporation, Cambridge, MA, USA) in trauma surgery and articular calcaneal fractures.[61,62] Calcaneal bone defects were filled with Biobon to augment internal fixation and were followed for 1 year. These studies showed that autogenous bone graft can be replaced by a resorbable calcium phosphate substitute for the use of filling bone voids and augmenting fixation. The bone substitute was biocompatible and resorbed within 6 months of implantation.

Clinical studies concluded that Norian SRS allowed earlier postoperative weight bearing without compromising scoring on a calcaneal scoring measure. Csizy and colleagues[63] provide a case report that describes the usefulness of Norian SRS in preserving Böhler's angle in a patient at 2 years under weight-bearing conditions. Despite this resistance to compression, little of the bone substitute had undergone osseous integration 2 years after implantation. Norian SRS is known to have a higher compressive strength than α-BSM (55 MPa vs 10–15 MPa), but it is absorbed less rapidly in vivo.[61,64,65]

Johal and colleagues[66] studied whether open reduction and internal fixation (ORIF) augmented with an injectable bioresorbable calcium phosphate paste (α-BSM) is superior to ORIF alone in the treatment of calcaneal bone voids encountered after operative treatment of displaced intraarticular calcaneal fractures. These investigators randomized 47 patients with 52 closed displaced intraarticular fractures. ORIF alone was performed for 28 fractures and/or ORIF augmented with calcium phosphate in 24. The maintenance of Böhler's angle was evaluated at follow-up visits for more than 1 year. Secondary outcome measures included the Short Form (36) Health Survey and lower extremity measure every 6 months, and the Oral Analog Scale score at 2 years. These results support the use of an injectable calcium phosphate paste that hardens in situ to fill the bone void after a displaced intraarticular calcaneal fracture. There was no effect on general health, limb-specific function, and pain past 2 years and no associated complications with α-BSM use, supporting its safety as an addition to ORIF. The results of this study show that use of α-BSM leads to less calcaneal collapse after operative management once weight bearing is begun. They suggest the use of a bioresorbable calcium phosphate paste to fill the cancellous bone defect and augment ORIF to support the articular surface after a displaced intraarticular calcaneal fracture.

TCP

One of the commonly available resorbable ceramics is TCP. TCPs may be produced by either a conventional high-temperature ceramic process by heating nonmetallic mineral salts at temperatures greater than 1000°C, a process known as sintering, or a low-temperature aqueous chemical method. Coralline ceramics are formed by thermochemically treating coral with ammonium phosphate, leaving TCP with a structure and porosity that are similar to those of cancellous bone. TCP $(Ca_3[PO_4]_2)$ bone graft substitutes are composed of 39% calcium and 20% phosphorus by weight, and they have a range of multidirectional interconnected pores. TCP can assume one of 2 crystalline structures: α-TCP has a polygonal shape, whereas β-TCP is spherical, has a higher porosity, and can be packed more densely in a bone defect. β-TCP has a finer microarchitecture, which results in a faster resorption rate than that of α-TCP.[47] Most commercially available TCP bone graft substitutes are of the β variety.

Unlike calcium phosphate cements, which are pastes, TCP is available in either granular or block form. The compressive and tensile strength of β-TCP is similar to that of cancellous bone.[41] It is brittle and weak under tension and shear forces. Tricalcium blocks are often used for noncontained defects. Because the compressive strength of both coralline hydroxyapatite and TCP is similar to that of cancellous bone, neither product is used in situations in which greater mechanical strength is required. TCP granules may be used as a bone graft extender.

TCP undergoes resorption by dissolution and fragmentation in 6 to 18 months.[67] Resorption of TCP occurs via osteoclasts without an inflammatory or giant cell response. The bone volume produced is always less than the volume of the TCP that is resorbed.[67]

Cameron[68] evaluated the incorporation time of TCP by placing an 8.5- by 3-mm disk of the material into the cut surface of tibiae in a series of 20 patients undergoing total knee replacement. The disks of TCP could not be detected radiographically at 6 months, and the investigators concluded that TCP was a useful resorbable bone filler material.

In a retrospective case series, 43 patients with traumatic bone defects or nonunion of the femur, tibia, calcaneus, humerus, ulna, or radius had treatment augmented with TCP. Ninety percent of the fractures and 85% of the nonunions had united at the time of follow-up, at an average of 12 months (minimum duration, 6 months). The investigators concluded that TCP was a useful substitute for cancellous bone.[69]

Composite Graft

Although most of the initial experimental and clinical work has been performed with products used in isolation as a single variable, these products may have qualities that are mutually beneficial when used in combination. Therefore, different combinations continue to be explored.

Calcium sulfate + calcium phosphate

One concept of ideal synthetic bone void filler might combine the features of relatively rapid resorption of $CaSO_4$ with the slower resorption of calcium phosphates $(CaPO_4)$. The calcium sulfate in the composite graft resorbs early but the calcium phosphate takes 180 days for complete resorbtion. A $CaSO_4$-$CaPO_4$ composite graft material might enhance vascular infiltration and replacement of the graft by new bone, thus promoting improved restoration of a bone defect. Early start and a slow rate of absorption promotes bone formation into the bolus of cement, and a portion of calcium phosphate continues to provide a scaffold, which eventually is incorporated into new bone.[70]

Such a hybrid bone graft substitute in the form of a triphasic $CaSO_4$-based injectable composite that incorporates a matrix of calcium sulfate dihydrate and dicalcium phosphate dehydrate with β-TCP granules (PRO-DENSE, Wright Medical Technology Inc, Arlington, TN, USA) has been tested in an animal experiment. The injectable $CaSO_4$-$CaPO_4$ composite graft increased the amount and strength of restored bone when compared with conventional $CaSO_4$ pellets after 13 and 26 weeks in a canine critical-sized bone defect model and when compared with specimens of normal bone.[70]

This $CaSO_4$-$CaPO_4$ composite graft may be advantageous in the treatment of benign bone tumors and in trauma applications, including distal radius, tibial plateau, and vertebral compression fractures, or other settings in which an enhanced amount and strength of restored bone using a highly biocompatible bone graft substitute are desirable.

Such a composite graft in injectable form may also be used to increase purchase of hardware in osteoporotic bones in which bone failure, not implant breakage, is the primary mode of failure of internal fixation. Because bone mineral density correlates with the holding power of screws, osteoporotic bone often lacks the strength to hold plates and screws securely. Resistance to pull-out of a screw placed in bone depends on the length of the screw purchase, the thread of the screw, and the quality of the bone itself. A variety of substances have also been used to enhance screw purchase in bone, including bone auto- or allograft and bone cement. PMMA injection into the screw hole before pedicle screw insertion has been shown to dramatically improve axial pull-out resistance and the resistance to screw toggle caused by cyclic caudocephalic loading.[71,72] However, it is not commonly used clinically because of intraoperative and long-term problems, including the risk for neural injury, risk for thermal necrosis during polymerization, cement extrusion into fracture site and joint,[73,74] the toxicity of the polymerization reaction of PMMA,[75] and complications of revision surgery and hardware removal.[76,77] Furthermore, PMMA can physically block endosteal and periosteal new bone formation during fracture healing,[78] and PMMA evokes the formation of a fibrous membrane at the bone-cement interface, which produces several cytokines and inflammatory mediators that lead to bone resorption,[79–81] which is also caused by particulate PMMA wear debris.[82] Retained PMMA can act as a stress riser,[83] which increases the risk for refracture.

$CaSO_4$-$CaPO_4$ composite graft may be a better alternative to PMMA to inject in screw holes before inserting the screws to increase the purchase of hardware implanted. It is not associated with exothermic necrosis of adjacent tissues. It is biocompatible, bioresorbable, and osteoconductive, and thus has the potential for replacement by new bone during healing and normal bone turnover. A cadaver study compared purchase of the tibia pro fibula screws inserted at the level of the syndesmosis with and without augmentation of drill holes with injectable calcium sulfate. A statistically significant difference was noted in displacement, failure load, and failure energy between augmented and nonaugmented screws; the augmented screws were considerably stronger. The force necessary to pull out augmented screws was 100% to 200% greater than the force necessary to pull out nonaugmented screws. In nonaugmented screws, failure occurred through simple stripping of the bone at the bone-screw interface, and there were no instances of fibula fracture. In the augmented group, failure occurred through stripping of the screw-cement interface; the fibula fractured at the screw site in 50% of specimens. The pull-out resistance of augmented screws was such that failure occurred in the bone before the implant failed.[84]

Calcium phosphate + osteoinductive matrix
Another type of combination is a composite graft that attempts to accelerate bone formation by adding osteoinductive factors to the osteoconductive matrix of calcium

phosphate (Collagraft, Zimmer, Warsaw, IN, USA; Healos, Orquest, Mountain View, CA, USA). A prospective randomized multicenter trial comparing autogenous bone grafting to a composite graft of calcium phosphate matrix and bovine collagen with autogenous bone marrow as an adjunct in the treatment of long-bone fractures showed no significant difference in union rate, functional outcomes, or complications in 249 fractures (213 patients) over a 2-year follow-up. The investigators concluded that a calcium phosphate composite graft was as effective as an autogenous iliac crest bone graft for the treatment of long-bone fractures requiring bone graft augmentation. However, because few such fractures are routinely bone grafted and because there were no control patients without any grafting, the overall usefulness of the grafting was unknown (level I evidence).[85]

Calcium phosphate + recombinant human bone morphogenetic protein + polymers
Growth factors have been added to injectable calcium phosphate ceramics either before setting of the cement or after complete setting.[86,87] Because of the nonmacroporous structure of the calcium phosphate cement, one concern is that prolonged retention of entrapped proteins might result in the loss of their osteoinductive potential. If the recombinant human bone morphogenetic protein-2 (rhBMP-2) was loaded on a biodegradable polymer such as poly(DL-lactic-co-glycolic acid) and then combined with calcium phosphate, it would allow a controlled release of the growth factor from the microparticles, delivering a continuous level of bioactive protein to the surrounding tissues.

An in vitro study on release kinetics showed that incorporation of rhBMP-2-loaded microparticles in calcium phosphate cement results in a sustained release of rhBMP-2 under neutral and acidic conditions.[88] In an animal study, a single percutaneous injection of rhBMP-2–calcium phosphate matrix accelerated healing in nonhuman primate fibular osteotomy sites over a wide range of treatment times.[89]

SUMMARY

Multiple synthetic bone graft substitute options alone or in combination are available for use in patients to fill in a bone void caused by trauma or tumor, deliver high doses of antibiotics locally, improve purchase of hardware in osteoporosis, and accelerate healing. Although many of these products are used for similar indications, they differ considerably in their chemical composition, structural strength, and resorption or remodeling rates.

Most available studies are nonrandomized case series the efficacy of which cannot be proved. There is a lack of direct-comparison studies between different types of bone graft substitutes. Indiscriminate use without clear indications results in unnecessary financial costs. When used in the correct circumstance, bone graft substitutes improve patient outcomes by decreasing the loss of reduction of intraarticular fractures and improving bone formation and fracture healing in areas affected by trauma.

Future synthetic scaffold grafts offer the potential of performance superior to autograft because they can act as a scaffold for bone healing, be a source of mechanical stability, and if incorporated with bone induction factors provide stimulus for bone growth.

REFERENCES

1. Fleming JE Jr, Cornell CN, Muschler GF. Bone cells and matrices in orthopedic tissue engineering. Orthop Clin North Am 2000;31:357–74.
2. Stevenson S. Biology of bone grafts. Orthop Clin North Am 1999;30:543–52.

3. Banwart JC, Asher MA, Hassanein RS. Iliac crest bone graft harvest donor site morbidity. A statistical evaluation. Spine 1995;20:1055–60.

4. Hill NM, Horne JG, Devane PA. Donor site morbidity in the iliac crest bone graft. Aust N Z J Surg 1999;69:726–8.

5. Schnee CL, Freese A, Weil RJ, et al. Analysis of harvest morbidity and radiographic outcome using autograft for anterior cervical fusion. Spine 1997;22:2222–7.

6. Younger EM, Chapman MW. Morbidity at bone graft donor sites. J Orthop Trauma 1989;3:192–5.

7. Boyce T, Edwards J, Scarborough N. Allograft bone. The influence of processing on safety and performance. Orthop Clin North Am 1999;30:571–81.

8. Screening and testing of donors of human tissue intended for transplantation. Washington, DC: FDA, Center for Biologics Evaluation and Research; 1977.

9. Kagan RJ. Standards for tissue banking. McLean (VA): American Association of Tissue Banks; 1998.

10. Buck BE, Malinin TI, Brown MD. Bone transplantation and human immunodeficiency virus. An estimate of risk of acquired immunodeficiency syndrome (AIDS). Clin Orthop Relat Res 1989;240:129–36.

11. Delloye C, Hebrant A, Munting E, et al. The osteoinductive capacity of differently HCl-decalcified bone alloimplants. Acta Orthop Scand 1985;56:318–22.

12. Cornell CN, Lane JM. Current understanding of osteoconduction in bone regeneration. Clin Orthop Relat Res 1998;355(Suppl):S267–73.

13. Kühne JH, Bartl R, Frisch B, et al. Bone formation in coralline hydroxyapatite. Effects of pore size studied in rabbits. Acta Orthop Scand 1994;65:246–52.

14. Nakahara H, Goldberg VM, Caplan AI. Culture-expanded periosteal-derived cells exhibit osteochondrogenic potential in porous calcium phosphate ceramics in vivo. Clin Orthop Relat Res 1992;276:291–8.

15. Peltier LF, Jones RH. Treatment of unicameral bone cysts by curettage and packing with plaster-of-Paris pellets. J Bone Joint Surg Am 1978;60:820–2.

16. Yamamuro T. Bone bonding behavior and clinical use of A-W glass-ceramic. In: Urist MR, O'Connor BT, Burwell RG, editors. Bone grafts, derivatives and substitutes. Oxford (UK): Butterworth-Heinemann; 1994. p. 245–59.

17. Carson JS, Bostrom MP. Synthetic bone scaffolds and fracture repair. Injury 2007; 38(Suppl 1):S33–7.

18. Bohner M. Calcium orthophosphates in medicine: from ceramics to calcium phosphate cements. Injury 2000;31(Suppl 4):37–47.

19. Bauer TW, Smith ST. Bioactive materials in orthopaedic surgery: overview and regulatory considerations. Clin Orthop Relat Res 2002;395:11–22.

20. Bhattacharyya T, Tornetta P III, Healy WL, et al. The validity of claims made in orthopaedic print advertisements. J Bone Joint Surg Am 2003;85:1224–8.

21. Dreesmann H. Uber Knochenplombierung. Bietr Klin Chir 1892;9:804–10.

22. Peltier LF. The use of plaster of Paris to fill large defects in bone. Am J Surg 1959; 97:311–5.

23. Peltier LF. The use of plaster of Paris to fill defects in bone. Clin Orthop Relat Res 1961;21:1–31.

24. Gazdag AR, Lane JM, Glaser D, et al. Alternatives to autogenous bone graft: efficacy and indications. J Am Acad Orthop Surg 1995;3:1–8.

25. Mirzayan R, Panossian V, Avedian R, et al. The use of calcium sulfate in the treatment of benign bone lesions. A preliminary report. J Bone Joint Surg Am 2001;83:355–8.

26. Walsh WR, Morberg P, Yu Y, et al. Response of a calcium sulfate bone graft substitute in a confined cancellous defect. Clin Orthop Relat Res 2003;406: 228–36.

27. Sidqui M, Collin P, Vitte C, et al. Osteoblast adherence and resorption activity of isolated osteoclasts on calcium sulphate hemihydrate. Biomaterials 1995;16: 1327–32.
28. Bucholz RW. Nonallograft osteoconductive bone graft substitutes. Clin Orthop Relat Res 2002;395:44–52.
29. Turner TM, Urban RM, Gitelis S, et al. Radiographic and histologic assessment of calcium sulfate in experimental animal models and clinical use as a resorbable bone-graft substitute, a bone-graft expander, and a method for local antibiotic delivery: one institution's experience. J Bone Joint Surg Am 2001;83(Suppl 2[Pt 1]): 8–18.
30. Urban RM, Turner TM, Hall DJ, et al. Healing of large defects treated with calcium sulfate pellets containing demineralized bone matrix particles. Orthopedics 2003; 26(Suppl 5):s581–5.
31. Turner TM, Urban RM, Gitelis S, et al. Resorption evaluation of a large bolus of calcium sulfate in a canine medullary defect. Orthopedics 2003;26(Suppl 5): s577–9.
32. Kelly CM, Wilkins RW, Gitelis S, et al. The use of a surgical grade calcium sulfate as a bone graft substitute: results of a multicenter trial. Clin Orthop Relat Res 2001;382:42–50.
33. Hak DJ. The use of osteoconductive bone graft substitutes in orthopaedic trauma. J Am Acad Orthop Surg 2007;15:525–36.
34. Pietrzak WS, Ronk R. Calcium sulfate bone void filler: a review and a look ahead. J Craniofac Surg 2000;11:327–33.
35. Watson JT. The use of an injectable bone graft substitute in tibial metaphyseal fractures. Orthopedics 2004;27(Suppl 1):s103–7.
36. Borelli J Jr, Prickett WD, Ricci WM. Treatment of nonunions and osseous defects with bone graft and calcium sulfate. Clin Orthop Relat Res 2003;411:245–54.
37. Gitelis S, Piasecki P, Turner T, et al. The use of a calcium sulfate-based bone graft substitute for benign bone lesions. Orthopedics 2001;24:162–6.
38. Panchbhavi VK. Augmentation of internal fixation of osteoporotic ankle fracture using injectable bone substitute. Tech Foot Ankle Surg 2007;6:264–9.
39. McKee MD, Wild LM, Schemitsch EH, et al. The use of an antibiotic-impregnated, osteoconductive, bioabsorbable bone substitute in the treatment of infected long bone defects: early results in a prospective trial. J Orthop Trauma 2002;16:622–7.
40. De Long WG Jr, Einhorn TA, Koval K, et al. Bone grafts and bone graft substitutes in orthopaedic trauma surgery. A critical analysis. J Bone Joint Surg Am 2007;89: 649–58.
41. Frankenburg EP, Goldstein SA, Bauer TW, et al. Biomechanical and histological evaluation of a calcium phosphate cement. J Bone Joint Surg Am 1998;80: 1112–24.
42. Constantz BR, Ison IC, Fulmer MT, et al. Skeletal repair by in situ formation of the mineral phase of bone. Science 1995;267:1796–9.
43. Goodman SB, Bauer TW, Carter D, et al. Norian SRS cement augmentation in hip fracture treatment: laboratory and initial clinical results. Clin Orthop Relat Res 1998;348:42–50.
44. Jarcho M. Calcium phosphate ceramics as hard tissue prosthetics. Clin Orthop Relat Res 1981;157:259–78.
45. LeGeros RZ. Properties of osteoconductive biomaterials: calcium phosphates. Clin Orthop Relat Res 2002;395:81–98.
46. Knaack D, Goad ME, Aiolova M, et al. Resorbable calcium phosphate bone substitute. J Biomed Mater Res 1998;43:399–409.

47. Wiltfang J, Merten HA, Schlegel KA, et al. Degradation characteristics of α and β tri-calcium-phosphate (TCP) in minipigs. J Biomed Mater Res 2002;63:115–21.

48. Welkerling H, Raith J, Kastner N, et al. Painful soft-tissue reaction to injectable Norian SRS calcium phosphate cement after curettage of enchondromas. J Bone Joint Surg Br 2003;85:238–9.

49. Eriksson F, Mattsson P, Larsson S. The effect of augmentation with resorbable or conventional bone cement on the holding strength for femoral neck fracture devices. J Orthop Trauma 2002;16:302–10.

50. Desai BM. Osteobiologics. Am J Orthop (Belle Mead NJ) 2007;36(Suppl 4):8–11.

51. Cassidy C, Jupiter JB, Cohen M, et al. Norian SRS cement compared with conventional fixation in distal radial fractures. A randomized study. J Bone Joint Surg Am 2003;85:2127–37.

52. Hinz P, Wolf E, Schwesinger G, et al. A new resorbable bone void filler in trauma: early clinical experience and histologic evaluation. Orthopedics 2002;25(Suppl 5):s597–600.

53. Frayssinet P, Gineste L, Conte P, et al. Short-term implantation effects of a DCPD-based calcium phosphate cement. Biomaterials 1998;19:971–7.

54. Bajammal SS, Zlowodzki M, Lelwica A, et al. The use of calcium phosphate bone cement in fracture treatment. A meta-analysis of randomized trials. J Bone Joint Surg Am 2008;90:1186–96.

55. Benirschke SK, Sangeorzan BJ. Extensive intraarticular fractures of the foot. Surgical management of calcaneal fractures. Clin Orthop Relat Res 1993;292:128–34.

56. Sanders R. Displaced intra-articular fractures of the calcaneus. J Bone Joint Surg Am 2000;82:225–50.

57. Longino D, Buckley RE. Bone graft in the operative treatment of displaced intra-articular calcaneal fractures: is it helpful? J Orthop Trauma 2001;15:280–6.

58. Kiyoshige Y, Takagi M, Hamasaki M. Bone-cement fixation for calcaneus fracture–a report on 2 elderly patients. Acta Orthop Scand 1997;68:408–9.

59. Thordarson DB, Hedman TP, Yetkinler DN, et al. Superior compressive strength of a calcaneal fracture construct augmented with remodelable cancellous bone cement. J Bone Joint Surg Am 1999;81:239–46.

60. Schildhauer TA, Bauer TW, Josten C, et al. Open reduction and augmentation of internal fixation with an injectable skeletal cement for the treatment of complex calcaneal fractures. J Orthop Trauma 2000;14:309–17.

61. Bloemers FW, Stahl JP, Sarkar MR, et al. Bone substitution and augmentation in trauma surgery with a resorbable calcium phosphate bone cement. Eur J Trauma 2004;30:17–22.

62. Sarkar MR, Stahl JP, Wachter N, et al. Defect reconstruction in articular calcaneus fractures with novel calcium phosphate cement. Eur J Trauma 2002;28:340–8.

63. Csizy M, Buckley RE, Fennell C. Benign calcaneal bone cyst and pathologic fracture–surgical treatment with injectable calcium-phosphate bone cement (Norian): a case report. Foot Ankle Int 2001;22:507–10.

64. Larsson S, Bauer T. Use of injectable calcium phosphate cement for fracture fixation: a review. Clin Orthop Relat Res 2002;395:23–32.

65. Sarkar MR, Wachter N, Patka P, et al. First histological observations on the incorporation of a novel calcium phosphate bone substitute material in human cancellous bone. J Biomed Mater Res 2001;58:329–34.

66. Johal HS, Buckley RE, Le IL, et al. A prospective randomized controlled trial of a bioresorbable calcium phosphate paste (α-BSM) in treatment of displaced intraarticular calcaneal fractures. J Trauma 2009;67:875–82.

67. Moore WR, Graves SE, Bain GI. Synthetic bone graft substitutes. ANZ J Surg 2001;71:354–61.
68. Cameron HU. Tricalcium phosphate as a bone graft substitute. Contemp Orthop 1992;25:506–8.
69. McAndrew MP, Gorman PW, Lange TA. Tricalcium phosphate as a bone graft substitute in trauma: preliminary report. J Orthop Trauma 1988;2:333–9.
70. Urban RM, Turner TM, Hall DJ, et al. Increased bone formation using calcium sulfate-calcium phosphate composite graft. Clin Orthop Relat Res 2007;459:110–7.
71. Wittenberg RH, Lee KS, Shea M, et al. Effect of screw diameter, insertion technique, and bone cement augmentation of pedicular screw fixation strength. Clin Orthop Relat Res 1993;296:278–87.
72. Zindrick MR, Wiltse LL, Widell EH, et al. A biomechanical study of intrapeduncular screw fixation in the lumbosacral spine. Clin Orthop Relat Res 1986;203:99–112.
73. Harrington KD. The use of methylmethacrylate as an adjunct in the internal fixation of unstable comminuted intertrochanteric fractures in osteoporotic patients. J Bone Joint Surg Am 1975;57:744–50.
74. Bartucci EJ, Gonzalez MH, Cooperman DR, et al. The effect of adjunctive methylmethacrylate on failures of fixation and function in patients with intertrochanteric fractures and osteoporosis. J Bone Joint Surg Am 1985;67:1094–107.
75. Stürup J, Nimb L, Kramhøft M, et al. Effects of polymerization heat and monomers from acrylic cement on canine bone. Acta Orthop Scand 1994;65:20–3.
76. Wilkes RA, Mackinnon JG, Thomas WG. Neurological deterioration after cement injection into a vertebral body. J Bone Joint Surg Br 1994;76:155.
77. Kahanovitz N. Osteoporosis and fusion. Instr Course Lect 1992;41:231–3.
78. Yablon IG. The effect of methylmethacrylate on fracture healing. Clin Orthop Relat Res 1976;114:358–63.
79. Goldring SR, Schiller AL, Roelke M, et al. The synovial-like membrane at the bone-cement interface in loose total hip replacements and its proposed role in bone lysis. J Bone Joint Surg Am 1983;65:575–84.
80. Whitehill R, Stowers SF, Fechner RE, et al. Posterior cervical fusions using cerclage wires, methylmethacrylate cement and autogenous bone graft. An experimental study of a canine model. Spine 1987;12:12–22.
81. Whitehill R, Drucker S, McCoig JA, et al. Induction and characterization of an interface tissue by implantation of methylmethacrylate cement into the posterior part of the cervical spine of the dog. J Bone Joint Surg Am 1988;70:51–9.
82. Maloney WJ, Jasty M, Rosenberg A, et al. Bone lysis in well-fixed cemented femoral components. J Bone Joint Surg Br 1990;72:966–70.
83. Eschenroeder HC Jr, Krackow KA. Late onset femoral stress fracture associated with extruded cement following hip arthroplasty. A case report. Clin Orthop Relat Res 1988;236:210–3.
84. Panchbhavi VK, Vallurupalli S, Morris R, et al. The use of calcium sulfate and calcium phosphate composite graft to augment screw purchase in osteoporotic ankles. Foot Ankle Int 2008;29:593–600.
85. Chapman MW, Bucholz R, Cornell C. Treatment of acute fractures with a collagen-calcium phosphate graft material: a randomized clinical trial. J Bone Joint Surg Am 1997;79:495–502.
86. Lee DD, Tofighi A, Aiolova M, et al. α-BSM: a biomimetic bone substitute and drug delivery vehicle. Clin Orthop Relat Res 1999;367(Suppl):S396–405.
87. Blom EJ, Klein-Nulend J, Wolke JG, et al. Transforming growth factor-β1 incorporation in calcium phosphate bone cement: material properties and release characteristics. J Biomed Mater Res 2002;59:265–72.

88. Ruhe PQ, Hedberg EL, Padron NT, et al. rhBMP-2 release from injectable poly (DL-lactic-co-glycolic acid)/calcium-phosphate cement composites. J Bone Joint Surg Am 2003;85(Suppl 3):75–81.
89. Seeherman H, Li R, Bouxsein M, et al. rhBMP-2/calcium phosphate matrix accelerates osteotomy-site healing in a nonhuman primate model at multiple treatment times and concentrations. J Bone Joint Surg Am 2006;88:144–60.

Biologics in Foot and Ankle Surgery

Bryan J. Hawkins, MD

KEYWORDS

- Foot and ankle surgery • Biologics
- Bone morphogenetic proteins • Bone healing

Healing after bone injury or after arthrodesis is the result of a complex cascade of events. Autologous bone grafting is considered the "gold standard" intervention when fractures or fusions do not heal. The observation that healing could be successfully achieved after autologous grafting suggests that all of the factors required for healing are present in autologous bone. As a result of the work of Urist[1] beginning in 1965, the cascade of events that leads to bone healing is now understood. Urist[1] demonstrated that when the demineralized portion of autologous bone was implanted into the muscle of experimental animals, mature, new bone formed. The term applied to this process of causing ectopic bone to form is "osteoinduction." Further experimentation by Urist[1] and others ultimately led to the isolation of a family of proteins responsible for this process. These proteins were called bone morphogenetic proteins (BMP).

BMPs are endogenous proteins belonging to the transforming growth factor-β superfamily. Numerous BMPs have been isolated.[2] They are identified by number. BMP-2 and BMP-7 have the greatest osteoinductive capacity.[2,3] These proteins are important components of the healing cascade.

In basic terms, bone healing requires 3 components: osteoconductors, osteoinductors, and pluripotent mesenchymal stem cells. An osteoconductor is a scaffold over which new bone can form. Osteoinductors are proteins responsible for directing cellular differentiation into bone-forming cell lines; pluripotent mesenchymal stem cells are the target cells for the these proteins. An osteoconductor is either structural bone or a material that can serve as a base over which bone can form. In most circumstances, the osteoconductor is contained within the structure of a fracture or at the site of a fusion. In the circumstance where bone is missing and a gap or a void exists, an adequate scaffold may be absent. In these circumstances, an osteoconductor must be provided. Osteoconductors can be either bone material, whether autograft or allograft bone, or may in fact be composed of other materials that have osteoconductive characteristics, such as ceramics.

Although autologous bonegraft is the ideal graft material because it contains all of the material factors required for the healing cascade to proceed, its use has potential

Central States Ortho Specialists Inc, 6585 South Yale, Suite 200, Tulsa, OK 94136-8320, USA
E-mail address: bhawkins@csosortho.com

Foot Ankle Clin N Am 15 (2010) 577–596
doi:10.1016/j.fcl.2010.07.003
1083-7515/10/$ – see front matter © 2010 Elsevier Inc. All rights reserved.

limitations. The volume and quality of autologous bone available may be limited by the size and age of the patient and quantity may be further impaired because of previous surgery to harvest autologous graft.

Osteoinductive proteins are endogenous, but with the discovery of BMPs and the ability to manufacture them safely and cost effectively, the prospect of impacting the healing cascade by applying these proteins directly has become a reality. BMP-2 and BMP-7, the most potent osteoinductive proteins, have been manufactured using recombinant gene technology, such that they are available in high volume and concentration. BMP-2 is available as rhBMP2 Infuse Bonegraft (Medtronic, Memphis, TN, USA). Extensive study of the safety, toxicity, biocompatibility, and carcinogenicity of rhBMP2 Infuse Bonegraft preceded randomized human studies on its efficacy in anterior lumbar spinal fusion.[2] Favorable outcomes ultimately led to approval by the Food and Drug Administration (FDA) for the use of rhBMP2 Infuse Bonegraft for this indication.

It is reported that 6.2 million fractures occur in the United States per year with an estimated rate of delayed or nonunion ranging from 5% to 10%.[4] Failure rates of fusions are documented as well. Ankle arthrodesis failure rates are reported as high as 40%.[5] Studies of subtalar and midfoot fusion report failure rates of 16% to 30%.[6–8] Although it seems intuitive that rhBMP2 Infuse Bonegraft might be of value in the treatment of fracture or fusion nonunion, studies have focused more on its use in the spine. Its use was, however, evaluated in a prospective randomized study of 450 open fractures of the tibia of varying grades.[9] Patients were treated acutely with rhBMP2 Infuse Bonegraft as compared with standard treatment. The use of rhBMP2 Infuse Bonegraft resulted in more rapid healing with a significant decrease in the requirement for "additional" procedures. Its use was thus approved by the FDA for treatment of acute (within 14 days of injury) open fracture of the tibia treated with intra-medullary nail stabilization.

In addition to rhBMP2 Infuse Bonegraft, BMP-7 is available commercially (OP-1; Stryker Biotech, Hopkinton, MA). The clinical application of OP-1 was reviewed recently in the treatment of long bone nonunion. Giannoudis and colleagues[8] reported 100% healing in 45 patients with atrophic long bone nonunion treated with a regimen of autologous bone graft and OP-1. In another report, Moghaddam and colleagues[10] reported an 82% healing rate with the use of OP-1with and without autologous bone graft in a retrospective review of atrophic nonunions. Neither of these studies was controlled.

The decision to use an adjunctive osteoinductor resulted from two cases, established nonunions of the humerus and femur. Clinical considerations in each case precluded the use of autologous bone graft harvest in both cases. Rapid healing was noted in both of these original cases stimulating further interest in applying an osteoinductor in this manner. With the exception of two cases involving its use in acute open fractures of the tibia, the use of rhBMP 2 Infuse Bonegraft was "off label".

To date, no prospective, randomized clinical studies have been identified where the study premise involved the addition of an osteoinductor to produce healing in cases of established nonunion of either fractures or fusions. This review summarizes, retrospectively, the results of a large series of patients where rhBMP2 Infuse Bonegraft was utilized in cases of nonunion of the tibia, foot and ankle.

MATERIALS AND METHODS

From 2003 to the present, rhBMP2 Infuse Bonegraft was used in 101 cases. Data collection was maintained prospectively. Patients were evaluated clinically and radiographically. Time to healing was determined by a combination of clinical assessment of the resolution of symptoms and definitive radiographic healing either by standard radiographs or by computer-assisted tomography (CT). Aside from demographic considerations, patients were categorized as receiving adjunctive biologic grafting in either "primary" or "revision" situation, and in both the treatment of fractures and fusions. Treatment was considered primary if biologic implantation was used as part of the index procedure, either fracture treatment or fusion. Treatment was considered revision if the procedure using biologic implantation was done as a result of failure to achieve healing with at least one prior intervention for fracture or fusion. rhBMP2 Infuse Bonegraft was the only osteoinductive material used. If indicated, adjunctive osteoconductors were used.

The decision to use biologics was based solely on clinical judgment. The use of rhBMP2 Infuse Bonegraft in any revision setting seemed appropriate intuitively. Its use in a primary clinical setting was based on circumstances unique to each individual case. Many factors influenced the decision-making process. The most significant factors were comorbid medical conditions and the absence of available autologous graft. No specific guidelines were followed. All patients were counseled as to the proposed off-label use of rhBMP2 Infuse Bonegraft and consent for its use was obtained. No cases involved known infection or inflammatory arthritis.

Standard fracture or fusion stabilization was used. Revision of fixation using established principles was used when necessary. In the event of bone loss or void, an osteoconductive material was added. Autologous bonegraft (ABG) or tricalcium phosphate (TCP) (Matergraft, Medtronic, Memphis, TN, USA) was used when an osteoconductor was indicated. Results were analyzed, first by whether they were primary or revision procedures, then by the adjunctive grafting material used.

The decision to use rhBMP-2 Infuse was based on availability and the author's success with it prompted continued use of it. Its use was in the course of patient treatment and, as such, its use was not as a part of any study protocol. There were, therefore, no control study patients.

RESULTS
Overall

Of the 101 cases where rhBMP2 Infuse Bonegraft was used, 75 involved the tibia, foot, and ankle. Of the total, there were 40 female and 58 male patients with an age range of 18 to 78.One female patient underwent 2 separate grafting procedures and is considered as 2 separate case utilizations. One male patient had identical primary fusion on each foot at separate settings and is considered as 2 separate case utilizations, and another male patient underwent treatment for tibial nonunion in conjunction with an ipsilateral ankle arthrodesis, each considered as a separate case use. Of these, 61 involved the treatment of fractures (14 primary cases and 47 revision cases) and 40 involved the treatment of fusion (22 primary cases and 18 revision cases). Of these 101 cases, 87 healed, 7 failed to heal, 3 patients were lost to follow-up, and 4 patients are in active treatment at this time.

Tibia/Ankle/Foot

There were 75 cases involving the lower extremity below the knee (**Table 1**). Of these, 35 were fracture cases and 40 were fusion cases. Of the fusion cases, 22 were primary procedures and 18 were revisions of prior attempts at fusion. Of the fracture cases, 9 involved treatment of primary fracture and 26 involved the treatment of nonunion. There were 27 female and 44 male patients with an age range of 18 to 74 at the

Table 1
BMP patient database

NO	PT	DOB	Sex	FUS/FX	PRIM/REV	Side	Area	Location	DOS	TCP	ICBG	Healed?	Date Healed	Days	Weeks
1	KB	12/6/69	M	Fracture	Primary	L	Foot	5th MT	7/10/2007	No	No	Yes	02/22/08	227	32
2	RM	4/14/80	M	Fracture	Primary	L	Foot	Calcaneus	1/16/2007	Yes	No	Yes	04/07/07	81	12
3	LW	7/17/47	F	Fracture	Primary	R	Tibia	Distal	10/17/2008	No	No	Yes	02/09/09	115	16
4	BH	10/6/52	M	Fracture	Primary	L	Tibia	Distal	4/22/2008	Yes	No	Yes	06/11/08	50	7
5	MH	5/3/07	M	Fracture	Primary	L	Ankle	Distal	5/3/2007	Yes	No	Yes	07/24/07	82	12
6	SM	9/27/70	M	Fracture	Primary	L	Tibia	Shaft	8/11/2004	No	No	Yes	12/18/04	129	18
7	GR	2/1/69	F	Fracture	Primary	R	Tibia	Shaft	3/11/2008	No	No	Yes	06/30/08	111	16
8	JN	8/30/79	F	Fracture	Primary	L	Tibia	Shaft	12/5/2006	Yes	No	Yes	03/05/07	90	13
9	CJ	3/5/63	F	Fracture	Primary	R	Tibia	Shaft	7/12/2005	Yes	Yes	Yes	01/18/07	555	79
10	EC	3/1/45	F	Fracture	Revision	R	Foot	1st MT	12/29/2006	No	No	?	LTF		
11	AD	3/16/33	F	Fracture	Revision	L	Foot	1st MT	6/29/2004	No	No	Yes	09/15/04	78	11
12	JT	9/1/63	M	Fracture	Revision	L	Foot	5th MT	2/15/2008	No	No	Yes	05/06/08	81	12
13	RC	8/31/49	M	Fracture	Revision	L	Ankle	Bimalleolar	5/27/2008	No	No	Yes	08/06/08	71	10
14	RJ	9/4/70	M	Fracture	Revision	R	Tibia	Distal	6/3/2008	No	No	Yes	09/18/08	107	15
15	JS	12/31/73	M	Fracture	Revision	R	Tibia	Distal	4/22/2005	No	No	Yes	09/07/05	138	20
16	BC	6/13/56	M	Fracture	Revision	L	TIB/FIB	Distal	9/8/2006	Yes	No	Yes	12/20/06	103	15
17	JS	6/17/51	M	Fracture	Revision	R	TIB/FIB	Distal	3/25/2008	Yes	No	Yes	08/29/08	157	22
18	BH	10/23/91	M	Fracture	Revision	L	Tibia	PROX	8/15/2008	No	No	Yes	10/15/08	61	9
19	AH	7/2/46	M	Fracture	Revision	R	Tibia	PROX	1/8/2004	No	No	*No*			
20	DB	11/15/57	M	Fracture	Revision	L	Tibia	PROX	5/3/2006	No	Yes	Yes	06/26/06	54	8
21	DM	4/15/68	M	Fracture	Revision	R	Tibia	PROX	6/12/2009	No	Yes	Yes	10/26/09	136	19
22	SG	9/14/74	M	Fracture	Revision	R	Tibia	Shaft	7/28/2006	No	No	?	LTF		
23	BG	9/28/50	M	Fracture	Revision	L	Fibula	Shaft	8/23/2005	No	No	Yes	10/26/05	64	9
24	JJ	1/9/67	M	Fracture	Revision	L	Fibula	Shaft	3/29/2005	No	No	Yes	06/08/05	71	10
25	RG	6/12/89	M	Fracture	Revision	R	Fibula	Shaft	7/26/2007	No	No	Yes	10/08/07	74	11

26	GP	9/9/60	F	Fracture	Revision	L	Fibula	Shaft	12/12/2008	No	No	Yes	03/11/09	89	13
27	KP	9/6/73	F	Fracture	Revision	R	Fibula	Shaft	5/19/2005	No	No	Yes	08/20/05	93	13
28	VS	4/22/53	F	Fracture	Revision	L	Fibula	Shaft	1/11/2008	No	No	Yes	04/14/08	94	13
29	KL	9/30/53	M	Fracture	Revision	R	Tibia	Shaft	2/3/2005	No	No	Yes	09/30/05	239	34
30	TB	8/13/62	F	Fracture	Revision	L	Tibia	Shaft	11/13/2009	No	Yes	*Pending*			
31	SM	12/7/54	F	Fracture	Revision	R	Tibia	Shaft	10/31/2006	Yes	No	*No*			
32	RV	12/22/57	M	Fracture	Revision	L	Tibia	Shaft	1/14/2005	Yes	No	Yes	06/15/05	152	22
33	KR	11/14/64	F	Fracture	Revision	R	Tibia	Shaft	12/2/2008	Yes	Yes	Yes	03/09/09	97	14
34	CJ	3/5/63	F	Fracture	Revision	R	Tibia	Shaft	1/22/2006	Yes	Yes	Yes	03/05/07	407	58
35	TF	11/11/52	M	Fusion	Primary	L	Foot	1st TMT	5/18/2007	No	No	Yes	11/12/07	178	25
36	ED	7/7/48	F	Fusion	Primary	R	Foot	4/5 TMT Joint	3/27/2007	No	No	*No*			
37	KO	6/16/55	F	Fusion	Primary	R	Ankle	Joint	3/13/2007	No	No	Yes	07/19/07	128	18
38	JS	12/31/73	M	Fusion	Primary	R	Ankle	Joint	4/22/2005	No	No	Yes	09/07/05	138	20
39	JA	1/9/67	M	Fusion	Primary	L	Ankle	Joint	9/23/2005	No	No	Yes	02/20/06	150	21
40	PA	1/25/44	F	Fusion	Primary	R	Ankle	Joint	7/20/2006	No	Yes	Yes	11/20/06	123	18
41	RS	8/22/78	F	Fusion	Primary	L	Ankle	Joint	1/9/2009	No	Yes	Yes	05/21/09	132	19
42	DW	7/5/76	M	Fusion	Primary	R	Ankle	Joint	6/30/2009	Yes	Yes	*No*	10/21/09	113	16
43	RB	12/13/59	F	Fusion	Primary	R	Ankle	Joint	1/15/2010	No	Yes	*Pending*			
44	JS	3/14/61	M	Fusion	Primary	R	Foot	Lisfranc	8/24/2007	No	No	Yes	01/12/08	141	20
45	DL	10/7/54	M	Fusion	Primary	R	Foot	Subtalar	2/24/2009	No	No	Yes	05/04/09	69	10
46	DM	11/2/49	M	Fusion	Primary	L	Foot	Subtalar	3/13/2009	No	No	Yes	06/08/09	87	12
47	DM	12/24/64	M	Fusion	Primary	R	Foot	Subtalar	4/24/2007	No	No	Yes	08/02/07	100	14
48	RL	9/5/59	M	Fusion	Primary	L	Foot	Subtalar	1/19/2007	No	No	Yes	05/02/07	103	15
49	FF	5/16/66	M	Fusion	Primary	R	Foot	Subtalar	7/28/2006	No	No	Yes	11/13/06	108	15
50	RJ	9/4/70	M	Fusion	Primary	L	Foot	Subtalar	12/2/2008	No	No	Yes	04/22/09	141	20
51	LW	10/12/73	F	Fusion	Primary	R	Foot	Subtalar	6/19/2009	No	No	Yes	01/25/10	220	31
52	PH	6/21/72	M	Fusion	Primary	L	Foot	Subtalar	12/1/2006	No	No	Yes	12/07/07	371	53
53	RC	11/9/59	M	Fusion	Primary	R	Foot	T-N JOINT	12/9/2005	No	No	Yes	02/01/06	54	8

(continued on next page)

Table 1
(continued)

NO	PT	DOB	Sex	FUS/FX	PRIM/REV	Side	Area	Location	DOS	TCP	ICBG	Healed?	Date Healed	Days	Weeks
54	RC	11/9/59	M	Fusion	Primary	L	Foot	T-N JOINT	10/29/2004	No	No	Yes	01/13/05	76	11
55	CB	6/17/61	M	Fusion	Primary	L	Foot	T-N JOINT	4/7/2006	No	Yes	Yes	09/27/06	173	25
56	DM	9/23/72	F	Fusion	Primary	L	Foot	T-N JOINT	8/14/2007	Yes	No	Yes	01/14/08	153	22
57	LE	1/28/47	F	Fusion	Revision	L	Foot	1st TMT	4/29/2005	No	No	Yes	06/29/05	61	9
58	DP	2/17/49	F	Fusion	Revision	R	Foot	1st TMT	6/30/2009	No	No	Yes	10/19/09	111	16
59	CW	12/6/53	M	Fusion	Revision	L	Foot	2nd TMT	9/14/2004	No	No	Yes	11/22/04	69	10
60	JA	11/1/56	M	Fusion	Revision	L	Ankle	Distal	4/11/2006	Yes	No	Yes	11/28/06	231	33
61	JH	5/10/43	M	Fusion	Revision	R	Ankle	Joint	11/4/2005	No	No	Yes	02/22/06	110	16
62	EB	2/2/47	F	Fusion	Revision	L	Ankle	Joint	4/4/2006	No	Yes	Yes	09/11/06	160	23
63	DB	2/28/41	M	Fusion	Revision	R	Ankle	Joint	3/28/2008	No	Yes	Yes	09/28/08	184	26
64	VVW	8/25/40	M	Fusion	Revision	L	Ankle	Joint	10/19/2007	Yes	No	Yes	01/19/08	92	13
65	KH		F	Fusion	Revision	L	Ankle	Joint	2/20/2010	No	No	*Pending*			
66	TJ	3/30/60	M	Fusion	Revision	R	Foot	Lisfranc	10/22/2004	No	No	Yes	12/27/04	66	9
67	CL	2/25/60	F	Fusion	Revision	R	Foot	Lisfranc	2/17/2005	No	No	Yes	04/25/05	67	10
68	HE	6/4/32	M	Fusion	Revision	R	Foot	Subtalar	1/26/2006	No	No	Yes	04/13/06	77	11
69	JC	11/24/56	M	Fusion	Revision	R	Foot	Subtalar	6/11/2004	No	No	Yes	09/09/04	90	13
70	DL	8/22/58	M	Fusion	Revision	R	Foot	Subtalar	12/7/2007	No	No	Yes	03/11/08	95	14
71	FH	9/20/68	M	Fusion	Revision	L	Foot	Subtalar	9/16/2008	No	No	Yes	01/26/09	132	19
72	DP		F	Fusion	Revision	R	Foot	Subtalar	12/15/2009	No	No	*Pending*			
73	KS	6/25/56	F	Fusion	Revision	R	Ankle	TIB-CALC	6/30/2005	No	No	Yes	10/05/05	97	14
74	NL	1/21/49	F	Fusion	Revision	L	Foot	T-N JOINT	7/28/2009	No	Yes	Yes	11/01/09	96	14
75	JF	3/16/1990	M	Fracture	Revision	L	Foot	1st MT	7/2/2009	No	No	No	12/2/2009	153	22

Average weeks to healing = 43.2.
Range 7–79.

Abbreviations: DOB, date of birth; DOS, date of surgery; F, female; FUS/FX, fusion/fracture; ICBG, iliac crest bone graft; L, left; M, male; PRIM/REV, primary/revision; PT, patient; R, right; TCP, tricalcium phosphate; TMT, tarsometatarsal; T-N, talonavicular; LTF, Lost to followup; MT, metatarsal; TIB-CALC, tibiocalcaneal; PROX, proximal.

time of surgery. Of this group, 2 patients were lost to follow-up and 4 remain in active treatment, leaving 69 cases with final disposition.

Determination of time to healing was generally straightforward. In most cases, routine radiographs and clinical evaluation were sufficient to determine that healing had occurred. Other cases were not straightforward. If pain persisted, adjunctive CT scans were used to determine if bone healing had progressed or definitively occurred. In some cases (such as with segmental bone loss or nonunion of severe pilon fracture in a diabetic patient, as examples), the determination of healing was protracted. Patients were often protected for longer periods of time and adjunctive CT scanning was repeated at 90-day intervals to determine progress of healing.

The average time to healing for all 75 cases was 43.2 weeks (range 7.1–79.3). In a small number of cases, healing was protracted, increasing the average time to healing. We considered all cases in determining the average, but successful use does not necessarily imply complete healing. The following 2 examples illustrate, first, a case of complete straightforward healing, and a case of protracted healing with a second procedure necessary, but little doubt that the outcome was a clinical success.

In the first example, an isolated talonavicular fusion was performed in a 46-year-old male. Viewing radiographs, it appeared healed by 7 weeks (**Fig. 1**). In the second example, a 46-year-old female sustained segmental tibial bone loss (5 cm) after a severe open distal tibia fracture. After double plating and initial grafting, clear evidence of healing and consolidation occurred throughout the 5-cm area of bone loss. There remained questionable consolidation at the proximal junction of the bone-loss segment and the distal tibial shaft. Further grafting was recommended and ultimately this area of the defect was determined to be healed (**Fig. 2**). The first case demonstrates straightforward progression to healing, and the time to healing is easily determined. In the second example, significant healing occurred as the result of adjunctive grafting, but the healing was considered incomplete. After a second grafting procedure, complete healing was observed. It could be argued that this constituted a clinical failure once the requirement for additional grafting occurred. In this case, where the alternative is loss of the limb, both utilizations were considered a clinical success.

Because the use of rhBMP2 Infuse Bonegraft was determined to be in the best interest of the patient from clinical considerations alone, no protocol existed to govern its use. Patients fell into 3 treatment subsets. The first subset included those patients who had rhBMP2 Infuse Bonegraft used alone, the second were patients with rhBMP2 Infuse Bonegraft and ABG, and the third subset were patients who had rhBMP2 Infuse Bonegraft used with an osteoconductor, TCP (Mastergraft). These were not treatment arms in a study protocol so comparisons cannot be made among groups.

In the rhBMP2 Infuse Bonegraft alone group, 45 patients were determined to have healed and 1 patient did not heal. In the rhBMP2 Infuse Bonegraft with adjunctive ABG group, 8 patients demonstrated healing and 1 failed. In the group with rhBMP2 Infuse Bonegraft with adjunctive TCP, 12 patients demonstrated healing and 2 did not. The patient who did not heal in the rhBMP2 Infuse Bonegraft alone group was a 60-year-old female with a 20-year-old pantalar fusion. The patient developed severe tarsometatarsal (TMT) arthritis and fusion was attempted at the fourth/fifth TMT joint. In the group using rhBMP2 Infuse Bonegraft and adjunctive bone graft, the failure was in a proximal tibial fracture case in a diabetic patient. The failures in the rhBMP2 Infuse Bonegraft/TCP group involved a long-standing tibial shaft nonunion that failed to heal and a case of posttraumatic avascular necrosis (AVN) of the talus where attempted tibiotalar fusion failed (**Table 2**).

The use of rhBMP2 Infuse Bonegraft in the treatment of fusion was particularly encouraging. When used for subtalar fusion, either primary or revision, solid

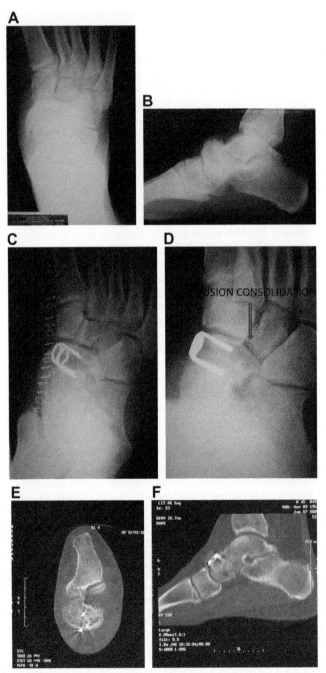

Fig. 1. (*A, B*) Preoperative radiographs of a 46-year-old male showing severe talonavicular degenerative arthritis. (*C, D*) Postoperative oblique radiographs of talonavicular fusion site: (*C*) immediate postoperative oblique; (*D*) 7-week oblique radiograph. (*E, F*) Axial and lateral CT images demonstrating consolidation of talonavicular fusion.

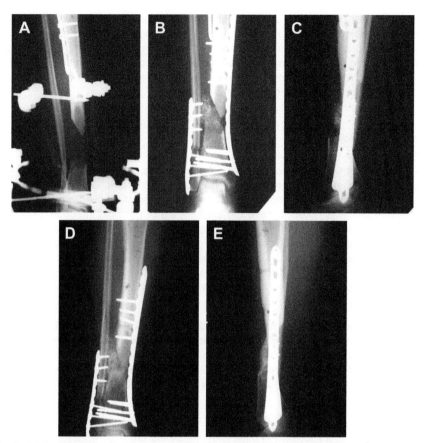

Fig. 2. (*A*) Radiograph of a 46-year-old female with segmental bone loss. (*B, C*) Anteroposterior (AP)/lateral radiographs 5 month after initial grafting. (*D, E*) Final AP/lateral radiographs 18 month after injury.

arthrodesis was achieved in all 9 cases. With the exception of the case of AVN of the talus, fusion was achieved in all ankle cases and in 5 cases of talonavicular arthritis, fusion, whether primary or secondary, was achieved in all cases.

The author did not attribute any complications such as wound breakdown, infection, or other local reactions such as increased redness or swelling to the use of rhBMP2

Table 2
Breakdown of infuse use with adjuncts (total = 68)

	Infuse Alone	Infuse with ABG	Infuse with TCP
Primary fracture	3	0	5
Primary fusion	16	3	2
Revision fracture	16	3	5
Revision fusion	11	3	2
Total	46	9	14

Abbreviations: ABG, autologous bonegraft; TCP, tricalcium phosphate.

Infuse Bonegraft. The author did see exuberant bone formation in certain cases and there was concern regarding its use in a periarticular location. In one case involving distal tibial application for a severely comminuted pilon fracture, joint stiffness was seen. This would have been expected given the severity of the initial injury. The author did not see significant heterotopic bone formation, nor was periarticular use associated with any specific intra-articular complications.

Case Presentations

Tibia

Case 1 Case 1 was a 44-year-old female, 1.5 years status post (s/p) intramedullary nail stabilization of a severely comminuted proximal tibia fracture. She presented with gross fracture motion, pain, and leg instability. At the time of initial surgical treatment, the fracture site was noted to have the appearance of possible infection. Definitive treatment was deferred after debridement for 6 weeks after cultures were positive. The patient underwent plate stabilization and grafting using Reamer/Irrigator/Aspirator System (Synthes, Paoli, PA, USA) graft harvest from the ipsilateral femur from a retrograde approach and rhBMP2 Infuse Bonegraft. Healing was deemed complete clinically and radiographically at 13.9 weeks. Initial and final radiographs are demonstrated in **Fig. 3**.

Case 2 A 25-year-old female who sustained bilateral tibia fractures in the left was comminuted/open. After initial irrigation and debridement with intramedullary nail stabilization, the patient underwent grafting for cortical bone loss at approximately 2 weeks. The defect was grafted with rhBMP2 Infuse Bonegraft and TCP (Mastergraft). Healing was deemed complete at 12.9 weeks. Initial and final radiographs are demonstrated in **Fig. 4**.

Ankle

Case 1 Case 1 was a 62-year-old male who underwent ankle arthrodesis with persistent joint line on x-ray and pain. The patient underwent revision fusion using rhBMP2 Infuse Bonegraft alone. The fusion site was determined to be stable and hardware was maintained at revision. Fusion was deemed complete at 15.7 weeks (**Fig. 5**).

Case 2 Case 2 was a 35-year-old male who sustained a severe intra-articular distal tibia fracture. The patient had a persistent fracture line extending up into the distal tibia and severe articular incongruity. The patient participated in heavy laboring work and requested amputation. It was suggested that attempts at salvage be undertaken. This would require both treatment for fracture nonunion and ankle arthrodesis. Blade plate stabilization achieved fixation for both the tibia and the ankle. The only adjunct used was rhBMP2 Infuse Bonegraft. Healing was deemed complete at 19.7 weeks. Preoperative and final radiographs are demonstrated in **Fig. 6**.

Case 3 A 67-year-old male with type 2 diabetes sustained a severely comminuted distal tibia fracture that evolved into a painful nonunion. There had been no apparent sepsis involved but severe venous insufficiency and compromised circulatory status were concerning. The recommendation was for strong consideration of below-knee amputation. Salvage was attempted after discussion of risks and that failure would warrant amputation. Retrograde imtramedullary nailing was accomplished with graft locally from morselized fibula and rhBMP2 Infuse Bonegraft. Consolidation was considered complete at 27 weeks. Preoperative and final radiographs are demonstrated in **Fig. 7**.

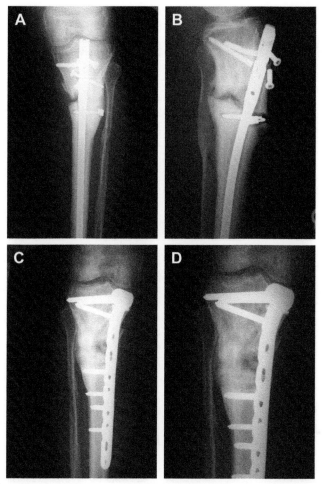

Fig. 3. (*A, B*) Radiographs of a 44-year-old female 17 months after open comminuted tibia fracture. (*C, D*) Fourteen weeks s/p bone graft with BMP-2.

Foot

Case 1 Case 1 was of a 60-year-old female who was 2.5 years s/p talonavicular fusion for painful degenerative joint disease. Radiographs revealed obvious nonunion. The patient underwent revision fusion with internal fixation, autologous bone graft, and rhBMP2 Infuse Bonegraft. Healing was considered complete at 14 weeks. Radiographs are demonstrated in **Fig. 8**.

Case 2 Case 2 was of a 19-year-old male with type 1 diabetes who sustained fractures of the first and second metatarsals of the left foot. He underwent open reduction internal fixation (ORIF) of both fractures. The second metatarsal fracture healed but the first metatarsal showed no healing after 11 months. He underwent an rhBMP-2 Infuse implantation of the first metatarsal. Bridging consolidation and clinical healing was deemed complete at 22 weeks (**Fig. 9**).

Case 3 Case 3 was of a 47-year-old male who sustained an open injection injury to the plantar aspect of his foot. Foreign material was injected into the foot and acute

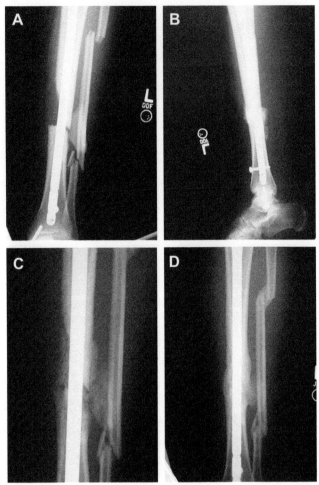

Fig. 4. (*A, B*) Radiographs of a 25-year-old female with s/p L open tibia fracture with cortical bone loss. (*C, D*) Postoperative AP views: (*C*) 10 weeks postoperative; (*D*) 16 weeks postoperative.

infection ensued. The injury included a comminuted fracture of the fifth metatarsal with cortical loss. After multiple debridements and clinical resolution of the infection, the patient underwent delayed primary ORIF of the fifth metatarsal fracture with implantation of rhBMP-2 Infuse Bonegraft. Serial radiographs demonstrating consolidation of the fracture are noted in **Fig. 10.**

DISCUSSION

The author's results using rhBMP2 Infuse Bonegraft have been very encouraging. Anecdotal experience must be supported, ultimately, by appropriately controlled, randomized study. The first premise of its use is that it seemed intuitive that adjunctive grafting with biologics would be beneficial in very challenging clinical circumstances. A randomized, controlled study involving this type of patient would be difficult to

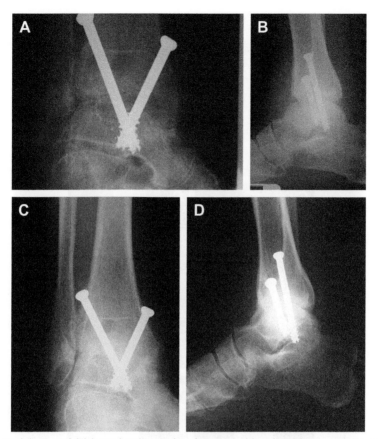

Fig. 5. AP (*A*) AP and (*B*) lateral radiographs of 62-year-old male with persistent nonunion of ankle arthrodesis. (*C, D*) Sixteen weeks after grafting with BMP-2 alone.

construct and enroll. A single fusion site such as the ankle or subtalar joint would provide for an adequate patient population with respect to potential enrollees. This could potentially be constructed as a revision study if enough numbers of nonunion cases could be identified.

The tibia presents a unique opportunity for study because it is commonly injured and larger numbers of tibial nonunions ultimately develop. Friedlander and colleagues[11] evaluated 122 patients with tibial pseudarthrosis who were treated with OP-1 (BMP-7) implantation and compared these patients with a control group who were treated with intramedullary nailing and autologous grafting. Healing rates were similar, actually slightly higher in the control group, but the difference was not statistically significant. When nicotine use was factored in, the OP-1 patients showed a higher rate of union. Other studies are being developed to use the tibial nonunion as the basis for a prospective randomized trial at this time.

Cost is a consideration for the use of any adjunctive treatment. Cost effectiveness may be a better focus of analysis rather than actual cost alone. Autologous bone harvest and grafting carries actual cost, as well as the potential cost of morbidity associated with it. In their study of open tibia fractures, Govender and colleagues[9] noted a significant reduction in the number of "additional" procedures, such as grafting,

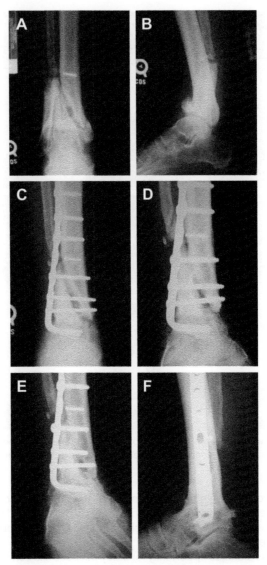

Fig. 6. (*A, B*) Radiographs of a 31-year-old male s/p intra-articular distal tibia fracture with nonunion and ankle arthrosis. (*C, D*) Postoperative AP radiographs of BMP-2 grafting of tibial nonunion and ankle arthrodesis: (*C*) 14 weeks posterative; (*D*) 19 weeks postoperative. (*E, F*) Final radiographs after 1 year.

debridement for infection, or hardware revision in the patients treated with rhBMP2 Infuse Bonegraft. In short, if a bone heals with the index intervention, there will be huge cost savings over the circumstance where it does not heal. Alt[12] assessed the costs incurred in treating Gustilo grade III open fractures of the tibia in the European health system. Social costs were estimated by considering the relationship between healing time (lost work productivity) as well as the cost of adjunctive procedures. The patients in whom rhBMP-2 was used incurred huge cost savings when all of these

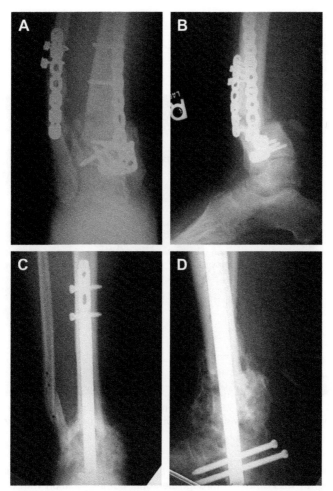

Fig. 7. (*A, B*) Radiographs of a 67-year-old male with type 2 diabetes mellitus 14 months after a severe pilon fracture with multiple interventions. (*C, D*) A 67-year-old male s/p intramedullary nail fusion for revision distal tibial nonunion with BMP-2 and local bone. Radiographs show AP and lateral fusion 28 weeks postoperative.

factors were taken into account. The front end cost of the BMP is negligible in comparison to the savings.

In addition to the optimum indications for the use of adjunctive biologics and the cost effectiveness of these treatment modalities, the actual "method" of application of the biologic protein at the time of surgery needs to be better clarified. rhBMP2 Infuse Bonegraft comes as powder that is reconstituted at the time of application to a liquid. The liquid is applied to an absorbable sponge consisting of bovine collagen. The protein adsorbs to the collagen after 15 minutes and is then contained at a concentration of 1.5 mg/mL. The sponge is then applied to the surgical site. In the author's experience, there are 2 "application" options: on lay or inlay. When one considers its use in a long bone, it may not be possible to apply the sponge "inside" the bone, so it is literally laid onto the bone and held in place by local tissue (muscle

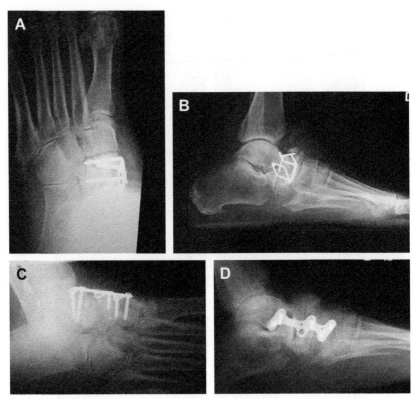

Fig. 8. (*A*, *B*) Radiographs of a 60-year-old female 28 months s/p talonavicular fusion with painful nonunion. (*C, D*) s/p revision fusion with BMP-2 and bone graft at 13 weeks.

and/or periosteum). Advice on the optimal application techniques in utilizing rhBMP2 Infuse Bonegraft was obtained through personal communication with other experienced practitioners. The recommendation was to contain the collagen sponge if at all possible. When revising a fusion nonunion, it is easy to see how containment is possible. In the case of revision ankle fusion, the author would actually create channels between the opposing fusion surfaces and contain the collagen sponges within this space. This is the same recommendation for subtalar fusions, where containment is relatively easy. This may explain why the author has seen such encouraging results in the treatment of failed arthrodesis of the ankle and subtalar joint.

When structural bone graft or TCP (Mastergraft) is used, the recommendation would be to roll or fold the collagen sponge around the graft material and then apply both to the surgical site. Oftentimes, the application of the biologic protein and the osteoconductor involved both inlay or containment of some of the material with on lay of the remaining material. The optimum application technique will hopefully be further elucidated with additional study.

No complications were attributable to the use of rhBMP2 Infuse Bonegraft. Numerous reports have outlined concerns with the use of rhBMP2 Infuse Bonegraft in the cervical spine.[13–15] These included both local reactions and heterotopic bone formation. Neurologic compromise has been attributed to the use of rhBMP2 Infuse Bonegraft in the lumbar spine.[16] In a recent study, the use of rhBMP2 Infuse Bonegraft

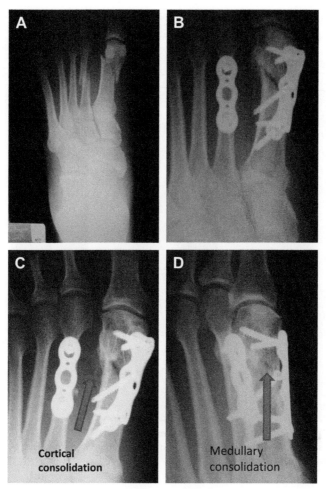

Fig. 9. (A, B) Radiographs of a 19-year-old male with type 1 diabetes: (A) AP radiograph of initial injury; (B) 11-month postoperative radiograph showing nonunion of first metatarsal fracture. (C, D) Final radiographs 4-months postoperative.

in the treatment of complex tibial plateau fractures demonstrated a significantly higher incidence of heterotopic bone formation in cases where rhBMP2 Infuse Bonegraft had been used. The heterotopic bone formed typically at the location of implantation and 4 of 17 patients underwent reoperation to remove the heterotopic bone.[12,17]

Very little literature addresses the use of biologic adjuvants in foot and ankle surgery. Bibbo and Haskell[18] reported early results of the addition of rhBMP2 Infuse Bonegraft in "high-risk" patients undergoing foot and ankle surgery. The "high-risk" status was determined by the presence of comorbid conditions such as diabetes and immunosuppression, among others. High rates of healing were seen in ankle and subtalar fusions at an average of 10 weeks.

The use of rhBMP2 Infuse Bonegraft in the treatment of difficult or failed fractures and fusions has been encouraging. Its use in 101 instances over a 7-year period points to very rare use. Most patients were selected for negative reasons. That is, other

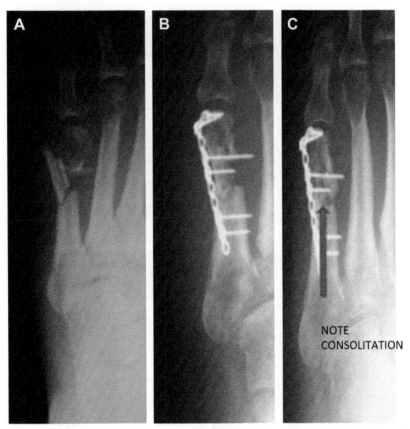

Fig. 10. (*A–C*) Radiographs of a 47-year-old male with comminuted open fracture of the fifth metatarsal. (*A*) AP radiograph of initial injury and (*B*) 1 month postoperative and (*C*) 6 months postoperative.

standard treatments were either not indicated or not available. Other cases were selected for the sheer difficulty expected with healing and the consequences if healing did not occur. Ten cases involved patients in whom amputation was the only other viable option, or would have been the option with another failure to heal. Limb salvage is preferable usually from a clinical standpoint, but also from the standpoint of cost effectiveness. Williams[19] estimated the lifetime prosthetic cost to exceed $400,000 in a small study of limb salvage patients with an average age of 41. The author would strongly consider the use of rhBMP-2 Infuse in any situation where limb salvage was dependent on fracture or fusion healing.

Some clinical situations appeared to respond differently to the use of rhBMP2 Infuse Bonegraft. Fusion healing occurred rapidly. Fracture healing was not as consistent or dramatic. In cases of atrophic long bone fractures, healing would occur rapidly in one case and would fail in another. This experience is not reflected in these data, as this involved the femur and humerus, but it is noteworthy. In addition, rhBMP2 Infuse Bonegraft cannot be used as the only adjunct when a void or defect exists. An osteo-conductor must be included in this circumstance and further study of the effects of different osteoconductive materials is warranted. Reviewing experience with atrophic fracture of the humerus, rapid healing was noted in the circumstance where a significant loss of cortical bone was present and adjunctive allograft bone chips were applied with the rhBMP2 Infuse Bonegraft. Complete absence of healing was noted in another case of well-fixed fracture without bone loss where rhBMP2 Infuse Bonegraft was the only adjunct used.

rhBMP2 Infuse Bonegraft was not used in any case involving Charcot neuroarthropathy of the foot. It was used in many diabetic patients, with success, after fracture, and in one instance of fusion in what was Charcot involvement of the ankle. rhBMP2 Infuse Bonegraft was not used in any case with known infection. It was utilized in one case after treatment of an infected nonunion of the tibia (Tibia case 1). In addition, it was used in a case of resolved septic arthritis of the ankle. In this case rhBMP2 Infuse Bonegraft was used in conjunction with compression external fixation and the fusion healed rapidly.

Well-constructed, controlled studies will be required to further clarify the place of rhBMP2 Infuse Bonegraft, as well as other adjuvants in the clinical treatment of bone and joint problems in the foot and ankle. Significant data exist to demonstrate that the use of rhBMP 2 Infuse Bonegraft is both efficacious and cost effective. The author's results in a community-based setting involving 101 cases (75 involving the lower extremity below the knee) suggest that the use of rhBMP 2 Infuse Bonegraft can positively affect the healing process in challenging clinical circumstances. Additional study will refine the indications for the use of biologic adjuvants, but the ability to influence the healing process in this manner is promising.

REFERENCES

1. Urist MR. Bone: formation by autoinduction. Science 1965;150:893–9.
2. Chen D, Zhao M, Mundy GR. Bone morphogenetic proteins. Growth Factors 2004;22:233–41.
3. Wozney JM, Rosen V. Bone morphogenetic protein and bone morphogenetic gene family in bone formation and repair. Clin Orthop Rel Res 1998;346:26–37.
4. Praemer A, Furner S, Rice DP, editors. Musculoskeletal conditions in the United States. Rosemont (IL): American Academy of Orthopedic Surgeons; 1999.
5. Frey C, Halikus HM, Vu-Rose T, et al. A review of ankle arthrodesis: predisposing factors to nonunion. Foot Ankle 1994;15:581–4.
6. Easley ME, Trnka HJ, Schon LC. Isolated subtalar arthrodesis. J Bone Joint Surg Am 2000;82:613–24.
7. Bibbo C, Anderson RB, Davis WH, et al. Complications of midfoot and hindfoot arthrodesis. Clin Orthop Rel Res 2001;391:45–58.
8. Giannoudis P, Kanakaris N, Dimitriou R, et al. The synergistic effect of autograft and BMP-7 in the treatment of atrophic nonunion. Clin Orthop Rel Res 2009; 467:3239–48.
9. Govender S, Csimma C, Genant HK, et al. Recombinant human bone morphogenetic protein-2 for treatment of open tibial fractures: a prospective, controlled, randomized study of 450 patients. J Bone Joint Surg Am 2002;84:2123–34.
10. Moghaddam A, Elleser C, Biglari B, et al. Clinical application of BMP-7 in long bone nonunions. Arch Orthop Trauma Surg 2010;130:71–6.
11. Friedlander GE, Perry CR, Cole JD, et al. Osteogenic protein-1 (bone morphogenetic protein-7) in the treatment of tibial nonunions. J Bone Joint Surg Am 2001; 83(Suppl 1):S151–8.
12. Alt V, Donnell S, Chhabra A, et al. A health economic analysis of the use of rhBMP-2 in Gustilo-Anderson grade III open tibial fractures for the UK, Germany and France. Injury 2009;40:1269–75.

13. Joseph V, Rampersaud YR. Heterotopic bone formation with the use of rhBMP-2 in posterior minimal access interbody fusion: a CT analysis. Spine 2007;32: 2885–90.
14. Perri B, Cooper M, Lauryssen C, et al. Adverse swelling associated with the use of rh-BMP-2 in anterior cervical discectomy and fusion: a case study. Spine J 2007;7:235–9.
15. Shields LB, Raque GH, Glassman SD, et al. Adverse effects with high-dose re-combinant human bone morphogenetic protein-2 use in anterior cervical spine fusion. Spine (Phila Pa 1976) 2006;31:542–7.
16. Wong DA, Kumar A, Jatana S, et al. Neurologic impairment from ectopic bone in the lumbar canal: a potential complication of off-label PLIF/TLIF use of bone morphogenetic protein-2 (BMP-2). Spine J 1988;242:1528–34.
17. Boraiah S, Paul O, Hawkes D, et al. Complications of recombinant human BMP-2 for treating complex tibial plateau fractures. Clin Orthop Rel Res 2009;467: 3257–62.
18. Bibbo C, Haskell MD. Recombinant bone morphogenetic protein-2 (rhBMP-2) in high risk foot and ankle surgery: surgical techniques and preliminary results of a prospective, intention to treat study. Tech Foot Ankle Surg 2007;6:71–9.
19. Williams MO. Long-term cost comparison of major limb salvage using the Ilizarov method versus amputation. Clin Orthop Rel Res 1994;301:156–8.

Autologous Bone Graft: When Shall We Add Growth Factors?

Peter V. Giannoudis, MB, MD, FRCS[a,b,*],
Haralampos T. Dinopoulos, MD[a]

KEYWORDS

• Nonunion • Bone defect • Autologous bone graft
• Growth factors • Graft expansion • BMPs

Despite the ongoing advances in the treatment of fractures and understanding of the fracture repair processes, impaired healing continues to be one of the most debilitating complications of fractures. Up to 10% of the 6.2 million fractures occurring annually in the United States are associated with impaired healing.[1] Many of these cases of impaired fracture healing demonstrate unique characteristics posed not only by the initial trauma sustained with bone defects and impaired vascularity of the area but also as a result of previous treatment modalities. Many of these patients require lengthy treatments associated with both functional and psychosocial impairment. Not less worthy is the economical burden to the patient and the health system.[2]

The standard treatment of most aseptic nonunions is mechanical stabilization with or without biologic stimulation depending on the assessment and classification of the nonunion.[3]

The current gold standard for any given situation requiring bone grafting and especially in situations of fracture nonunion is autologous bone grafting (ABG). Autologous cancellous bone grafting remains a unique biologic method promoting union by stimulating the local biology at the nonunion site.[4–7] Autologous bone has all three components necessary to promote or enhance bone regeneration: an osteoconductive scaffold, endogenous bioactive molecules, and cells that are able to respond to these signals. Unfortunately, although autogenous bone is considered as the best graft option, significant complications have been reported related to the harvesting site,

This article originally appeared in *Orthopedic Clinics of North America* 2010;41(1):85–94.
[a] Department of Trauma & Orthopedic Surgery, University of Leeds, Leeds General Infirmary, Great George Street, Leeds LS1 3EX, UK
[b] Academic Trauma & Orthopedic Unit, Floor A Clarendon Wing, Leeds General Infirmary University Hospital, Great George Street, Leeds LS1 3EX, UK
* Corresponding author. Academic Trauma & Orthopedic Unit, Floor A Clarendon Wing, Leeds General Infirmary University Hospital, Great George Street, Leeds LS1 3EX, UK.
E-mail address: pgiannoudi@aol.com

most often being the anterior iliac crest of the pelvis.[8] Furthermore, the desirable quantity of the required graft at times may be insufficient.[8]

For these reasons, over the years other biologically based strategies have been developed. These include electrical, ultrasound, and shockwave stimulation, a wide range of bone graft substitutes with either osteoconductive or both osteo-conductive and osteoinductive properties, and biologic response modifiers that are administered either locally or systemically, including bone morphogenetic proteins (BMPs), platelet-derived growth factors, and parathyroid hormone.[9–11] These bio-logic response modifiers, appear to have been used successfully in managing nonunions.[12–14] In addition to nonunion, the administration of these molecules has been used in many other orthopedic situations, including stabilization of implants,[15,16] restoration of large segmental bone defects,[15,17] treatment of osteo-necrosis of the femoral head,[18] fusion of joints, cartilage regeneration,[19,20] augmentation of periprosthetic fractures, and acceleration of fracture healing, especially in patients at high risk of fracture nonunion.[21]

Nonetheless, there are still adverse clinical settings where despite providing the best mechanical environment modification complemented with ABG, failure has occurred.[22–27] In addition, there are circumstances where the application of growth factors in isolation would not seem enough to promote successful bone healing.[28]

In this study, therefore, we consider in what clinical situations implantation of autol-ogous bone grafting may need enhancement with commercially available growth factors (BMP-2 and BMP-7) to promote successful bone healing.

THE USE OF AUTOLOGOUS BONE GRAFTING OR REAMING BY-PRODUCTS

Tibia is the most common long bone to sustain a fracture. It has a high risk of devel-oping nonunion because of the compromised soft tissue envelope especially over its anterior medial area.[25,29] Consequently, it represents the bone with the highest overall incidence of nonunion, and the "nonunion model."[25]

In the atrophic nonunions, the biologic factor is considered to be mostly the problem, despite the perception that the vascularity at the nonunion site is not compromised. The oligotrophic and even more the atrophic nonunions present insuf-ficient blood supply, or insufficient quantities of bone-forming cells. As a result, augmentation of this poor biologic environment through graft expansion is considered mandatory in achieving union in these difficult nonunion cases.[27,30–34] Several reports exist in the literature illustrating the efficacy of autologous iliac crest bone graft (AICBG) in isolation but also in combination with other materials. Overall the success rate with AIGBG is approximately 80% to 90%.[35–42]

The biologic properties of the "by-products" of reaming (RBP) have gained special interest very early in the history of reamed intramedullary nailing (IMN), representing an internal autografting procedure during closed reamed nailing.[17,43–45] IMN and reaming offers the unique biomechanical advantages of an intramedullary splinting fixation, in association with the osteoinductive stimulus of the "by-products" of reaming.[23,44–46] The vascular flow between endosteum and periosteum of the long bones retains nutri-tion and healing of the nonunion sites even after the temporary destruction of the endosteal blood flow until it is restored.[47] Although it is debatable in the literature whether to perform the IMN procedure openly or closed, it seems that surgeons open the nonunion site in those cases where the existing hardware needs to be removed, in cases with severe malalignment, and in those cases where additional bone graft needs to be added owing to massive bony defects.[43,48–53] Reckling and Waters[54] reported favorable results in the series of 33 noninfected tibial nonunions that were treated with a posterolateral approach and cortico-cancellous bone application. On an average of 5 months solid healing was noted in 94% of the patients.

Megas and colleagues[53] treated 50 cases of aseptic tibial nonunions with reamed interlocking nail. On average the reamed IMN was performed 15.6 months post injury. Various primary fixation methods were used and 36% had been open fractures. A closed IMN was attempted in all cases, but in 16 an open procedure was finally performed because of irreducible malalignment or for removal of previous hardware. Autologous cancellous graft was added in three cases because of the extent of the bone deficit. All fractures united in a 6-month period post nailing and the method was advocated as highly effective and safe for aseptic tibial nonunions.

In 1999, Wu and colleagues[55] evaluated 25 cases of tibia shaft aseptic nonunions treated with exchange nailing. Most (88.9%) of the original fractures were closed, stabilized with dynamic nails and developed atrophic nonunions. Exchange nailing was performed without opening the nonunion site and the success rates were significant (96%) in an average period of 16 weeks.

In 2003, Wu presented another series[56] of treating tibial aseptic nonunions with reamed IMN. In this study the original fixation method was plating and in 28 cases with adequate follow-up progressed to union. On average, the nonunions healed in 4.5 months (3.0–7.5) after removal of the original plate fixation, excessive reaming of the medullary canal, and insertion of a Kuntscher nail (13 cases) or locked gerhard küntscher (GK) nail (15 cases). However, the author suggested that whenever a large bony defect is present there should be additional bone grafting from the lilac crest and not performing excessive reaming of the medullary canal.

In the series of Devnani,[24] long-bone fracture nonunions were treated with compression plate fixation and AICBG. Among them the author evaluated the time to union of 10 tibial aseptic nonunions, 8 atrophic and 2 hypertrophic. All of the tibial nonunions of this series united at an average of 19.8 weeks, with a satisfactory functional outcome.

A comparative study of Johnson and Marder for tibial aseptic nonunions treated with IMN was published in 1987.[50] The authors used open IMN techniques and compared the effect on healing rates of bone grafting the nonunion site with the byproducts of reaming, or with AICBG. Eleven atrophic and 11 hypertrophic cases were evaluated. Successfully treated were 20 nonunion sites (91.9%), with an average time to union of 12.5 weeks. A statistically significant difference between the atrophic and hypertrophic cases (14.4 vs 10.6 weeks, respectively) was identified. The authors compared their results with those of closed IMN techniques and identified major differences in the time to union in favor of their own open nailing techniques.

Sledge and colleagues[51] have described their experience with static reamed IMN for a period of 6 years. Forty aseptic tibial nonunions were treated with reamed arbeitsgemeinschaft für osteosynthesefragen (AO) or GK nails. The original injury in 18 of them was an open fracture and opening of the fracture site was used in 27 (67.5%) of them for removal of implants, proper realignment, and also for AICBG enhancement. The average time to union was 7.1 months (12–67) and the union rates were 100%. No statistically significant differences were observed between open or closed IMN techniques and the use or not of AICBG for enhancement.

An overview of articles with the proven value of AICBG and RBPs is presented in **Table 1**.

THE USE OF GROWTH FACTORS

Aiming to overcome the limitations of the autologous bone grafting, bone morphogenetic proteins (BMP-7 and BMP-2) were produced by recombinant DNA

Table 1
Articles referring to union rates of fractures enhanced either with iliac crest autologous graft or with reamed–by products

Author Year	Anatomic Site	Method	Graft Used	Results/Union Rates
Reckling & Waters 1980[54]	Tibial 11 closed # 22 open #	Plaster	33 ICAG	93.9%
Johnson & Marder 1987[50]	Tibial treatment nonunion fractures	22 tibial # 8 closed # 11 open # (All open # IMN)	10 ICAG 12 RBP	90.9%
Sledge et al 1989[51]	40 tibial #s 18 closed # 22 open #	13 AO nails 27 GK nails 13 closed 27 open	10 ICAG 40 RBP	100%
Wiss et al 1992[30]	50 tibial #s 4 closed 46 open	All compression plating	39 ICAG	96%
Wiss & Stetson 1994[23]	47 tibial #s 14 closed 33 open	IMN	47 RBP	89%
Wu et al 1999[55]	25 closed #s	Reamed IMN	25 RBP	96%
Devnani 2001[24]	10 tibial #s 3 closed 7 open	All compression plating	10 ICAG	100%
Friedlaender et al 2001[12]	124 tibial #s 53 closed 71 open	Locked IMN	61 ICAG 63 BMP-7	62% vs 74%
Megas et al 2001[53]	50 tibial #s 32 closed # 18 open #	GK reamed IMN 34 closed technique 16 open	50 RBP 3 ICAG	100%
Wu 2003[56]	28 tibial #s 25 closed # 3 open #	13 GK 15 Kuntscher all open	28 RBP	100%

Abbreviations: BMP, bone morphogenetic protein; ICAG, iliac crest autologous graft; IMN, intramedullary nailing; RBP, reamed by-products.

technology.[57,58] They are substances with great osteoinductive properties for the enhancement of bone regeneration in various clinical applications, including the treatment of fracture nonunions.[8,59,60] The safety of their administration, combined with the lack of morbidity and the quantity restrictions that characterize autologous bone grafts, have given to this family of molecules a principal role over the other bone graft substitutes.[22]

The initial experimental in vivo and vitro work on BMPs opened the way for the study of Friedlaender and colleagues that started in 1992 and published in 2001.[12] In their milestone work, they evaluated the application of rhBMP-7 (recombinant human bone morphogenic protein-7 or OP1) in tibial nonunions. One hundred and twenty-four tibia aseptic nonunions were enrolled in a multicenter randomized prospective controlled trial. Either rhBMP-7 (in 63 nonunions) or autologous bone graft (in 61 nonunions) was used for enhancement of nonunion healing. The method of fixation was IMN for all cases (locked in 92%). At 9 months postsurgery, 62% of the rhBMP-7 group and 74% of the AICBG group demonstrated radiological union (P = .158). Overall, the rhBMP-7 administration was safe and proved to be statistically comparable to the gold standard biologic enhancement of autograft. This randomized trial of Friedlaender and colleagues[12] has established BMPs as a bone graft option (see **Table 1**).

The work of Cook[61] (animal model) showed the efficacy of recombinant human osteogenic protein-1 in healing 2-cm segmental defects in nonhuman primates (in ulnae and tibia), whereas the controls filled with AICBG showed only little new bone formation.

This ability of BMPs to regenerate new bone was used in various situations. Following the work of Friedlaender and colleagues the tibia per se is the first model for clinical investigation of potential application of the BMPs.[12] They have been associated with augmenting standard fixation and grafting methods in the acute setting of fractures as well as in established nonunions.[12,21]

Lately, the use of BMPs enhanced with autologous grafting is emerging in literature in various adverse scenarios (**Table 2**).

In a multicenter registry and database (six university centers) observational study, Kanakaris and colleagues[62] focused on the application of BMP-7/OP-1. They presented the preliminary results, of a prospective case series of aseptic tibial nonunions. Sixty-eight patients fulfilled the inclusion criteria for this observational study, with a minimum follow-up of 12 months. The median duration of tibial nonunion before BMP-7 application was 23 months (range 9–317). Patients had undergone a median of 2 (0–11) revision procedures before the administration of BMP-7. In 41%, the application of BMP-7 was combined with revision of the fixation at the nonunion site. In 25 cases (36.8%), the BMP-7 was expanded with the use of autologous bone graft (AICBG), out of which 14 (56%) had been previously treated unsuccessfully with ABG. Nonunion healing was verified in 61 (89.7%) of 68 in a median period of 6.5 months (range 3–15).

Ronga and colleagues,[63] in an observational, retrospective, nonrandomized study on the use of BMP-7, reported on treating nonunions in various anatomic sites. The work was performed by the BMP-7 Italian Observational Study (BIOS) Group. The clinical series included 105 patients. Additional grafts were used based on the surgeon's decision. Radiographic and clinical assessments were performed at progressive time intervals on two groups: BMP-7 + autograft (A) or BMP-7 alone (B). The mean follow-up was 29.2 months. The last assessment showed an overall 88.8% success rate with an average healing time of 7.9 months. In complicated cases, the success of the BMP-7 + autograft group reached 83.3% compared with 76.5% of the standalone BMP-7. If fewer than three operations preceded, healing was 90.6% compared with 87.8% (BMP-7), and if more than 3 operations preceded, the success dropped to 77.8% compared with 75.0% of BMP-7. At 9 months there was overlapping between the unions recorded in the two groups with healing rates of 86.0% and 85.7%, respectively. This is an observational study that illustrates the efficacy of BMP-7 with and without bone grafting for the treatment of long bone nonunions. This type of observation is confirmed by the comparison of the results between the BMP-7 alone group and the BMP-7 + autograft group. The increase in the percentage rate of consolidations at different follow-up shows that the interval between 6 and 9 months is a period that can still be considered useful before declaring failure of the treatment. The overlapping of the results according to the variables "previous complications and number of previous operations" confirms the efficacy of BMP-7.

Dimitriou and colleagues[64] in their recent study evaluated the efficacy and safety of recombinant bone morphogenetic protein-7 (rhBMP-7 or OP-1) as a bone-stimulating

Table 2
Articles referring to union rates of fractures enhanced with growth factors

Authors	Anatomic Site	Graft Used	Results	Comments
Vaccaro et al 2003[28]	Posterolateral lumbar fusions No instrumentation	rhBMP-7 (OP-1) + ICAG	- 6/11 pts (55%) with radio-graphic solid fusion (study criteria) - 10/11 pts (91%) bridging bone on the AP film	Pilot safety and efficacy study of rhBMP-7 (OP-1)
Dimitriou et al 2005[64]	26 persistent upper and lower limb atrophic nonunions	- 17 (65.4%) ABG + rhBMP-7, - 1 (3.8%) case Freeze Dried Allograft + rhBMP-7	- 16/17 (94.1%) clinical & radiological union - only rhBMP-7 8/9 (88.9%) union	Persistent long-bone atrophic nonunions
Ronga et al 2006[63]	105 patients - 69 lower limp - 36 upper limp	38 only BMP-7 - 11 with an osteoconductive - 50 with ABG - 6 composite graft	90.6% (<2 operations) 77.8% (>3 operations)	Observational, retrospective, nonrandomized (BMP-7 Italian Observational Study [BIOS] Group)
Kanakaris et al 2008[62]	68 tibial aseptic nonunions 41% revision of the fixation 26 (38.2%) ORIF; 7 (10.3%) IMN; 6 (8.8%) Ex Fix	BMP-7/OP-1 in all Graft expansion with autograft 25, 36.8%	61 (89.7%)	Multicenter registry and database (6 University centers) observational study

Abbreviations: ABG, autologous cancellous bone graft; AP, anteroposterior; BMP, bone morphogenetic protein; Ex-Fix, external fixator; ICAG, iliac crest autologous graft; IMN, intramedullary nailing; ORIF, open reduction internal fixation; rhBMP-7, recombinant human bone morphogenic protein-7 or OP1.

agent in the treatment of persistent fracture nonunions. Twenty-five patients with 26 fracture nonunions were treated with rhBMP-7. There were 10 tibial nonunions, 8 femoral, 3 humeral, 3 ulnar, 1 patellar, and 1 clavicular nonunion. The mean follow-up was 15.3 months. The mean number of operations performed before rhBMP-7 application was 3.2, with autologous bone graft and bone marrow injection being used in 10 cases (38.5%). Both clinical and radiological union occurred in 24 (92.3%) cases, within a mean time of 4.2 months and 5.6 months, respectively. No complications or adverse effects from the use of rhBMP-7 were encountered. In 17 (65.4%) cases the BMP application was combined with AICBG. In 16 of these 17 cases nonunion healing was noted. From those who had only rhBMP-7 applied, 8 of 9 healed. Their study supports the view of application of rhBMP-7 combined with autologous bone grafting for the treatment of persistent fracture nonunions.

Vaccaro and colleagues[28] in a pilot safety and efficacy study examined rhBMP-7 (OP-1) as an adjunct to iliac crest autograft in posterolateral lumbar fusions. They combined OP-1 putty with autograft for intertransverse process fusion of the lumbar spine in patients with symptomatic spinal stenosis and degenerative spondylolisthesis following spinal decompression. Twelve patients underwent laminectomy and partial or complete medial facetectomy as required for decompression of the neural elements followed by intertransverse process fusion by placing iliac crest autograft and OP-1 putty between the decorticated transverse processes. No instrumentation was used. Patients were followed clinically using the Oswestry scale and radiographically using static and dynamic radiographs to assess their fusion status. Radiographic outcome was compared with a historical control (autograft alone fusion without instrumentation for the treatment of degenerative spondylolisthesis). The results showed 9 (75%) of the 12 patients obtained at least a 20% improvement in their preoperative Oswestry score, whereas 6 (55%) of 11 patients with radiographic follow-up achieved a solid fusion by the criteria used in this study. Bridging bone on the anteroposterior film was observed in 10 (91%) of the 11 patients. No systemic toxicity, ectopic bone formation, recurrent stenosis, or other adverse events related to the OP-1 putty implant were observed. A successful fusion was observed in slightly over half the patients in this study, using stringent criteria without adjunctive spinal instrumentation. This study did not demonstrate the superiority of OP-1 combined with autograft over an autograft alone historical control, in which the fusion rate was approximately 55%.

DISCUSSION

Autogenous bone grafting, usually derived from the iliac crest, is frequently used in the treatment of fracture nonunions. The donor-site morbidity and potentially limited supply of suitable autogenous bone are commonly recognized drawbacks. The proven value of reaming by-products, an internal autografting, is quite often inadequate to overcome adverse local circumstances.

Regardless of the ongoing developments of new approaches or the improvement of the current ones for the treatment of fracture nonunions, their management continues to be difficult, even for the more experienced orthopedic surgeons. In addition, there other orthopedic situations dealt in the acute setting or in a more chronic base, where the use of the AICBG alone seems inadequate to overcome the difficulties posed by the local environment. Union rates of different types of nonunions, different degrees of the magnitude of the initial injury, the extent of time between initial injury and final intervention, individual characteristics, multiple previous interventions, and diversities on the application of each biologic enhancement make comparisons and conclusions difficult. On the other hand, recent studies advocated the benefit and safety of rhBMP-7 or rhBMP-2 in several anatomic sites in nonunions.[13,62,63] Most of the work with BMPs is done on the aseptic long bone nonunion model. It is of interest, however, that recently Chen and colleagues[65] have shown that osteogenic protein-1 (BMP-7) can stimulate new bone formation in the presence of bacterial infection in an intramuscular osteoinduction model in the rat. They speculated that BMPs could eventually be considered as a treatment option to stimulate fracture healing even in the presence of infection and a fixation device and, therefore, earlier removal of the implant and a more timely and effective treatment of the infection could be feasible.

Dimitriou and colleagues[64] have shown 92.3% healing success in 24 of 26 persistent long bone nonunions with the use of graft expansion in these difficult scenarios. Accordingly, Ronga and colleagues[63] in their observational study gave an overall 88.8% healing rate, which showed to be influenced by the number of complications or the number of previous operations (subgroups), once again giving useful information for suggestion of graft expansion in those recalcitrant nonunions. On the contrary, the work of Vaccaro and colleagues[28] in spinal fusion applying the concept of graft expansion without instrumentation shows low healing rates and thus creates considerable skepticism. Nonetheless, the local spinal environment and the lack of instrumentation may explain the differences noted.

The addition of growth factors in AICBG as a graft expansion technique can be considered in situations where the local environment is not favorable for healing. In those situations, this approach of providing a power biologic stimulus in terms of osteogenicity, osteoconductivity, and osteoinductivity appears to be desirable especially in cases after an already failed autografting procedure for the treatment of fracture nonunions.[63,64] **Table 3** shows the properties of AICBG and BMPs. This approach could not only lower the average number of operations performed but also hospital stay and cost.[2,66] Another scenario for graft expansion with growth factors would be the fracture site with bone loss either circumferentially or as a length defect in the acute setting of trauma or during the aftermath treatment of a nonunion. When a long bone nonunion has been treated with intramedullary nailing in association with a significant bone defect at the nonunion site, the graft expansion principle should be considered. Seemingly, bone defects secondary to extensive debridement, fracture malalignment, or at a later stage (eradication of deep infection, excision of the nonunion site) where an open procedure is about to be performed, represents another potential indication for the concept of graft expansion. Another situation where expansion in the form of percutaneous BMP administration can be considered is a closed exchange nailing procedure for an oligotrophic nonunion where the reaming by-products do not seem adequate as internal grafting to promote healing. In case of serious bone loss, the use of bone graft is an obligatory surgical step.[62–64] However, the number of previous surgical interventions, the extent of the damage to the soft tissue, and the type of previous complications could assist the surgeon toward the choice of the use of autograft in association with BMPs or other biologic active substances and/or implantation of osteoprogenitor cells.

Another area of interest for consideration for graft expansion is the docking site during bone transfer (distraction osteogenesis procedures). Giotakis and colleagues,[66] with regard to the issue of the use of bone graft at the docking site, comment that "if surgeons are asked if bone grafts are used at the docking site, answers will vary from 'never' to 'always.' This is truer in cases with severe soft tissue damage and atrophic docking ends. However, it is the author's experience that a 'wait and see' approach to docking sites invariably produces extended periods of fixator use, sometimes exceeding the period needed for a regenerate column to consolidate. Nevertheless, bone grafts are not always necessary if docking site clearance and

---

Table 3
Properties and consideration of issues for use: autologous cancellous bone graft (ABG) versus bone morphogenetic proteins (BMPs)

Autologous Cancellous Bone Graft	Bone Morphogenetic Proteins
• Biologic method	• Lesser grafting strength compared with ABG
• Osteoconductivity (scaffold)	• Nonbiologic method
• Osteoinductivity	• Osteoinduction
• Viable mesenchymal cells	• No osteoconductivity
• Requires 2nd operation (harvest site)	• No cells
• Limited availability	• Easy of use
• Donor site morbidity	• Ample quantity
	• No donor site morbidity
	• No side effects
	• More expensive

> **Box 1**
> **Suggestions for graft expansion with growth factors in various adverse situations**
>
> 1. Bone loss at the time of injury.
>
> 2. Persistent nonunions, when AICBG has failed.
>
> 3. Significant bone defect at the nonunion site (>2 cm).
>
> 4. More than two previous surgical interventions, extensive damage to the soft tissues, and increased severity of previous complications
>
> 5. Presence of bone defect greater than 2 cm after extensive debridement, either initially (open injuries, highly comminuted fractures) or at a later stage (eradication of deep infection, excision of the nonunion site).
>
> 6. Exchange nailing to enhance the by-products (injection) especially if the nailing technique was open.
>
> 7. Fusion of joints where a defect is substantial and the quantity of AICBG is not sufficient.

preparation produces two coapted surfaces with contact over a large surface area. Only if contact is poor, bone grafts are mandatory." The possible use of BMPs remains to be seen along with the recreation of the "fresh fracture" at the docking ends.

In **Box 1**, we summarize the possible suggestions for graft expansion with growth factors in various adverse situations.

Regarding the economical burden, Dahabreh and coworkers[2] in a cost analysis of treatment of persistent fracture nonunions, compared the cost implications of treatment of persistent fracture nonunions before and after application of recombinant human BMP-7. Of 25 fracture nonunions, 9 were treated using BMP-7 alone and 16 using BMP-7 and bone grafting. As a final phase of their treatment, the patients were grafted with BMP-7 in all cases, and additional autograft was used in 64%. They concluded that the mean number of procedures per fracture performed before application of BMP-7 was 4.16, versus 1.2 thereafter. The overall cost of treatment of persistent fracture nonunions with BMP-7 was 47.0% less than that of the numerous previous unsuccessful treatments ($P = .001$). They concluded that the early BMP-7 administration in complex or persistent fracture nonunions could reduce significantly the overall cost of treatment.

The same investigation group more recently did a comparative analysis of the cost of treatment of tibial nonunions with either BMP-7 or AICBG. The authors reported that the average cost of treatment with BMP-7 was 6.78% higher ($P = .1$) than with AICBG, and most of this (41.1%) was related to the actual price of the BMP-7. In addition to the satisfactory efficacy and safety of BMP-7 in comparison with the gold standard of AICBG, as documented in multiple studies, its cost effectiveness was advocated favorably in this study.

In conclusion, the combined used of AICBG with growth factors (BMPs) can be considered as a powerful biologic stimulus for the treatment of several clinical case scenarios. Certain criteria should be considered for the use of this strategy and for justification of the potential financial implications.

REFERENCES

1. Praemer A, Furner S, Rice DP. Musculoskeletal injuries. In: Barnes, Noble, editors. Musculoskeletal conditions in the United States. Park Ridge (IL): American Academy of Orthopaedic Surgeons; 1992. p. 85–124.

2. Dahabreh Z, Dimitriou R, Giannoudis PV. Health economics: a cost analysis of treatment of persistent fracture non-unions using bone morphogenetic protein-7. Injury 2007;38(3):371–7.

3. Brinker MR. Nonunions: evaluation and treatment. In: Browner BD, Jupiter JB, Levine AM, et al, editors. 3rd edition. Skeletal Trauma Basic science management and reconstruction, vol. 1. Philadelphia: Saunders; 2003. p. 507–604.

4. Blick SS, Brumback RJ, Lakatos R, et al. Early prophylactic bone grafting of high-energy tibial fractures. Clin Orthop Relat Res 1989;(240):21–41.

5. Heiple KG, Goldberg VM, Powell AE, et al. Biology of cancellous bone grafts. Orthop Clin North Am 1987;18(2):179–85.

6. Johnson KD. Management of malunion and nonunion of the tibia. Orthop Clin North Am 1987;18(1):157–71.

7. Jones CB, Mayo KA. Nonunion treatment: iliac crest bone graft techniques. J Orthop Trauma 2005;19(Suppl 10):S11–3.

8. Younger EM, Chapman MW. Morbidity at bone graft donor sites. J Orthop Trauma 1989;3:192–5.

9. Cook SD, Wolfe MW, Salkeld SL, et al. Effect of recombinant human osteogenic protein-1 on healing of segmental defects in non-human primates. J Bone Joint Surg Am 1995;77(5):734–50.

10. Paterson DC, Lewis GN, Cass CA. Treatment of delayed union and nonunion with an implanted direct current stimulator. Clin Orthop Relat Res 1980;148:117–28.

11. Schaden W, Fischer A, Sailler A. Extracorporeal shock wave therapy of nonunion or delayed osseous union. Clin Orthop Relat Res 2001;387:90–4.

12. Friedlaender GE, Perry CR, Cole JD, et al. Osteogenic protein- 1 (bone morphogenetic protein-7) in the treatment of tibial nonunions: a prospective, randomized clinical trial comparing rhOP-1 with fresh bone autograft. J Bone Joint Surg Am 2001;83:151–8.

13. Giannoudis PV, Tzioupis C. Clinical applications of BMP-7: the UK perspective. Injury 2005;36(Suppl 3):S47–50.

14. Johnson EE, Urist MR, Finerman GA. Resistant nonunions and partial or complete segmental defects of long bones. Treatment with implants of a composite of human bone morphogenetic protein (BMP) and autolyzed, antigen-extracted, allogeneic (AAA) bone. Clin Orthop Relat Res 1992;277:229–37.

15. Cook SD, Barrack RL, Patron LP, et al. Osteogenic protein-1 in knee arthritis and arthroplasty. Clin Orthop Relat Res 2004;428:140–5.

16. Zhang R, An Y, Toth CA, et al. Osteogenic protein-1 enhances osteointegration of titanium implants coated with periapatite in rabbit femoral defect. J Biomedical Materials Res Part B Appl Biomaterials 2004;71(2):408–13.

17. Mont MA, Jones LC, Elias JJ, et al. Strut-autografting with and without osteogenic protein-1: a preliminary study of a canine femoral head defect model. J Bone Joint Surg Am 2001;83(7):1013–22.

18. Lieberman JR, Conduah A, Urist MR. Treatment of osteonecrosis of the femoral head with core decompression and human bone morphogenetic protein. Clin Orthop Relat Res 2004;429:139–45.

19. Boden SD, Martin GI Jr, Morone MA, et al. Posterolateral lumbar intertransverse process spine arthrodesis with recombinant human bone morphogenetic protein 2/hydroxyapatitetricalcium phosphate after laminectomy in the nonhuman primate. Spine 1999;24(12):1179–85.

20. Cook SD, Dalton JE, Tan EH, et al. In vivo evaluation of recombinant human osteogenic protein (rhOP-1) implants as a bone graft substitute for spinal fusions. Spine 1994;19(15):1655–63.

21. Govender S, Csimma C, Genant HK, et al. BMP-2 Evaluation in Surgery for Tibial Trauma (BESTT) Study Group. Recombinant human bone morphogenetic protein-2 for treatment of open tibial fractures: a prospective, controlled, randomized study of four hundred and fifty patients. J Bone Joint Surg Am 2002;84(12): 2123–34.
22. Phieffer LS, Goutet JA. Delayed unions of the tibia. Instr Course Lect 2006;55: 389–401.
23. Wiss DA, Stetson WB. Tibial nonunion: treatment alternatives. J Am Acad Orthop Surg 1996;4(5):249–57. ·
24. Devnani AS. Simple approach to the management of aseptic non-union of the shaft of long bones. Singapore Med J 2001;42(1):20–5.
25. Souter WA. Autogenous cancellous strip grafts in the treatment of delayed union of long bone fractures. J Bone Joint Surg Br 1969;51(1):63–75.
26. Rodriguez-Merchan EC, Gomez-Castresana E. Internal fixation of nonunions. Clin Orthop Relat Res 2004;419:13–20.
27. Stevenson S. Enhancement of fracture healing with autogenous and allogeneic bone grafts. Clin Orthop Relat Res 1998;355(Suppl):S239–46.
28. Vaccaro AR, Patel T, Fischgrund J, et al. A pilot safety and efficacy study of OP-1 putty (rhBMP-7) as an adjunct to iliac crest autograft in posterolateral lumbar fusions. Eur Spine J 2003;12(5):495–500.
29. Schmidt AS, Christopher G, Finkemeier CG, et al. Treatment of closed tibial fractures. J Bone Joint Surg Am 2003;85(2):352–68.
30. Wiss DA, Johnson DL, Miao M. Compression plating for non-union after failed external fixation of open tibial fractures. J Bone Joint Surg Am 1992;74(9): 1279–85.
31. Weber BG, Brunner C. The treatment of nonunions without electrical stimulation. Clin Orthop Relat Res 1981;161:24–32.
32. La Velle DG. Delayed union and nonunion of fractures. In: Terry Canale S, editor. 9th edition. Campbell's operative orthopaedics, 2. St Louis (MO): Mosby; 1998. p. 579–629.
33. Gershuni DH, Pinsker R. Bone grafting for nonunion of fractures of the tibia: a critical review. J Trauma 1982;22(1):43–9.
34. Boskey AL, DiCarto E, Paschatis E, et al. Comparison of mineral quality and quantity in iliac crest biopsies from high- and tow-turnover osteoporosis: an FTIR microspectroscopic investigation. Osteoporos Int 2005;16(12):2031–8.
35. Heckman JD, Ehter W, Brooks BP, et al. Bone morphogenetic protein but not transforming growth factor-beta enhances bone formation in canine diaphyseal nonunions implanted with a biodegradable composite polymer. J Bone Joint Surg Am 1999;81(12):1717–29.
36. Trueta J. Blood supply and the rate of heating of tibial fractures. Clin Orthop Relat Res 1974;105:11–26.
37. Reed AA, Joyner CJ, Brownlow HC, et al. Human atrophic fracture non-unions are not avascular. J Orthop Res 2002;20(3):593–9.
38. Reed AA, Joyner CJ, Isefuku S, et al. Vascularity in a new model of atrophic nonunion. J Bone Joint Surg Br 2003;85(4):604–10.
39. Bruder SR, Fink DJ, Captan AI. Mesenchymal stem cells in bone development, bone repair, and skeletal regeneration therapy. J Cell Biochem 1994; 56(3):283–94.
40. Marsh JL, Buckwalter JA, McCollister-Evarts C. Delayed union, non-union, malunion and avascular necrosis. In: Epps Chang L, editor. Complications in orthopaedic surgery. 3rd edition. Philadelphia: JB Lippincott; 1994. p. 183–211.

41. Mohan S, Baylink D. Chapter 80. Principles of bone biology 1996;11:11–23.
42. Ring D, Barrick WT, Jupiter JB. Recalcitrant nonunion. Clin Orthop Relat Res 1997;340:181–9.
43. Christensen NO. Kuntscher intramedullary reaming and nail fixation for non-union of fracture of the femur and the tibia. J Bone Joint Surg Br 1973;55(2):312–8.
44. Danckwardt-Lilliestrom G. Reaming of the medullary cavity and its effect on diaphyseal bone. A fluorochromic, microangiographic and histologic study on the rabbit tibia and dog femur. Acta Orthop Scand Suppl 1969;12:81–153.
45. Olerud S, Kartstrom G. Secondary intramedullary nailing of tibial fractures. J Bone Joint Surg Am 1972;54(7):1419–28.
46. Reichert IL, McCarthy ID, Hughes SP. The acute vascular response to intramedullary reaming. Microsphere estimation of blood flow in the intact ovine tibia. J Bone Joint Surg Br 1995;77(3):490–3.
47. Utvag SE, Grundnes O, Reikeras O. Graded exchange reaming and nailing of non-unions. Strength and mineralisation in rat femoral bone. Arch Orthop Trauma Surg 1998;118(1–2):1–6.
48. Clancey GJ, Winquist RA, Hansen ST Jr. Nonunion of the tibia treated with Kuntscher intramedullary nailing. Clin Orthop Relat Res 1982;167:191–6.
49. Kempf I, Grosse A, Rigaut P. The treatment of noninfected pseudarthrosis of the femur and tibia with locked intramedullary nailing. Clin Orthop Relat Res 1986; 212:142–54.
50. Johnson EE, Marder RA. Open intramedullary nailing and bone-grafting for non-union of tibial diaphyseal fracture. J Bone Joint Surg Am 1987;69(3): 375–80.
51. Sledge SL, Johnson KD, Henley MB, et al. Intramedullary nailing with reaming to treat non-union of the tibia. J Bone Joint Surg Am 1989;71(7):1004–19.
52. Wiss DA, Stetson WB. Nonunion of the tibia treated with a reamed intramedullary nail. J Orthop Trauma 1994;8(3):189–94.
53. Megas P, Panagiotopoulos E, Skrivitiotakis S, et al. Intramedullary nailing in the treatment of aseptic tibial nonunion. Injury 2001;32(3):233–9.
54. Reckling FW, Waters CH. Treatment of non-unions of fractures of the tibial diaphysis by posterolateral cortical cancellous bone-grafting. J Bone Joint Surg Am 1980;62(6):936–41.
55. Wu CC, Shih CH, Chen WJ, et al. High success rate with exchange nailing to treat a tibial shaft aseptic nonunion. J Orthop Trauma 1999;13(1):33–8.
56. Wu CC. Reaming bone grafting to treat tibial shaft aseptic nonunion after plating. J Orthop Surg (Hong Kong) 2003;11(1):16–21.
57. Johnson EE, Urist MR, Finerman GA. Bone morphogenetic protein augmentation grafting of resistant femoral nonunions. A preliminary report. Clin Orthop Relat Res 1988;230:257–65.
58. Ozkaynak E, Rueger DC, Drier EA, et al. OP-1 cDNA encodes an osteogenic protein in the TGF-beta family. EMBO J 1990;9(7):2085–93.
59. Arrington ED, Smith WJ, Chambers HG, et al. Complications of iliac crest bone graft harvesting. Clin Orthop Relat Res 1996;329:300–9.
60. Fernyhough JC, Schimandle JJ, Weigel MC, et al. Chronic donor site pain complicating bone graft harvesting from the posterior iliac crest for spinal fusion. Spine 1992;17(12):1474–80.
61. Cook SD. Preclinical and clinical evaluation of osteogenic protein-1 (BMP-7) in bony sites. Orthopedics 1999;22(7):669–71.
62. Kanakaris NK, Calori GM, Giannoudis PV, et al. Application of BMP-7 to tibial non-unions: a 3-year multicenter experience. Injury 2008;39(S2):S83–90.

63. Ronga M, Baldo F, Zappala G, et al. Recombinant human bone morphogenetic protein-7 for treatment of long bone non-union: an observational, retrospective, non-randomized study of 105 patients. Injury 2006;37(Suppl 3):S51–6.
64. Dimitriou R, Dahabreh Z, Katsoulis E, et al. Application of recombinant BMP-7 on persistent upper and lower limb nonunions. Injury 2005;36(Suppl 4):S51–9.
65. Chen X, Kidder LS, Schmidt AH, et al. Osteogenic protein-1 induces bone formation in the presence of bacterial infection in a rat intramuscular osteoinduction model. J Orthop Trauma 2004;18(7):436–42.
66. Giotakis N, Narayan B, Nayagam S. Distraction osteogenesis and nonunion of the docking site: Is there an ideal treatment option? Injury 2007;38:S100–7.

Stem Cells in Bone Grafting: Trinity Allograft with Stem Cells and Collagen/Beta-Tricalcium Phosphate with Concentrated Bone Marrow Aspirate

Gregory P. Guyton, MD, Stuart D. Miller, MD*

KEYWORDS

- Bone graft • Trinity allograft • Beta-tricalcium phosphate
- Mesenchymal stem cells

The orthopedic foot and ankle surgeon needs bone grafts in the clinical situation of fracture healing and in bone-fusion procedures. Although the need for graft remains controversial for some procedures such as triple arthrodesis, many surgeons prefer to augment bone-on-bone healing with biology as well as to fill the gaps or "dead space" left after some procedures. The need for some sort of graft with traumatic cavitation or fracture comminution warrants even further merit. Frank nonunions or resection of bone, such as for avascular necrosis, infection, or tumor, provide uncontroversial need for bone graft filling. This article briefly outlines thought processes and techniques for 2 recent options for the surgeon. The Trinity product is a unique combination of allograft bone and allograft stem cells. The beta-tricalcium phosphate and collagen materials provide an excellent scaffold for bone growth; when combined with concentrated bone marrow aspirate they also offer osteoconductive and osteoinductive as well as osteogenerative sources for new bone formation.

Department of Orthopaedic Surgery, Union Memorial Hospital, 3333 North Calvert Street, Suite 400, Baltimore, MD 21218, USA
* Corresponding author.
E-mail address: smiller@gcoa.net

Foot Ankle Clin N Am 15 (2010) 611–619
doi:10.1016/j.fcl.2010.09.003
1083-7515/10/$ – see front matter © 2010 Published by Elsevier Inc.

foot.theclinics.com

PART I. TRINITY EVOLUTION AS AN ALLOGRAFT AUGMENTATION

Trinity Evolution (Orthofix International NV, Boston, MA, USA) is a proprietary allograft formulation specifically created to contain 3 separate elements to induce bone healing. These include:

1. Living osteogenic cells (both mature osteoblasts and osteoprogenitor cells)
2. An osteoconductive matrix
3. Osteoinductive cytokines.

The material is essentially a mixture of a consistent and very high concentration of mesenchymal stem cells, a fine cancellous bone matrix, and an admixture of demineralized cortical bone. In concept, osteogenesis, osteoconductivity, and osteoinduction are supplied by the 3 components respectively.[1]

GRAFT HANDLING

The graft itself is processed sterilely from the donor and the mesenchymal stem cell component is concentrated by a proprietary process. It can be stored on site after shipping at −70°C to −80°C for up to 3 months and must be used immediately once thawed. Thawing is accomplished in the operating room at a temperature no greater than 39°C to avoid cellular necrosis. A fluid component is present in the preparation including dimethyl sulfoxide (DMSO) cryoprotectant and the mesenchymal stem cell–specific basal medium. This is decanted after thawing immediately before implantation (**Fig. 1**). The thawing protocol must be followed precisely, as loss of stem cell viability may otherwise result.

MESENCHYMAL STEM CELLS IN HUMAN USE

Mesenchymal stem cells (MSCs) are a population of adult mesenchymal cells that can initiate a differentiation pathway into multiple different connective and bony tissues. Multiple roles for MSCs in vivo have been described, including serving as progenitor cells for bone remodeling and repair,[2] cartilage formation,[3] vascular support,[4] hematopoietic support,[5] and as progenitors for adipocytes.[3] MSCs have been proposed for a role in a variety of human tissue engineering applications, including the treatment of nonunions or supporting healing in high-risk fusion procedures.

Recent data suggest that MSCs naturally occur as perivascular cells (formerly called "pericytes") that are released at zones of injury. Activated MSCs then secrete large amounts of trophic and immunomodulatory cytokines. The trophic characteristics stimulate the tissue angiogenesis critical for healing as well as simulator local tissue progenitor cells. The resultant healing tissue, then, is primarily the result of the activation of the healing process of the surrounding tissue rather than directly derived from the MSCs themselves.[6]

MSCS AS AN ALLOGRAFT

The immunomodulatory cytokines are particularly important. They inhibit host lymphocyte surveillance of the injured tissues and prevent a large-scale autoimmune response.[1] The immunomodulatory characteristics of MSCs allows for the use of cells of allogeneic origin. Even the use of xenograft-sourced MSCs has been explored. Culture-expanded MSCs do not appear to elicit a significant host immune response even when directly infused intravenously.[7]

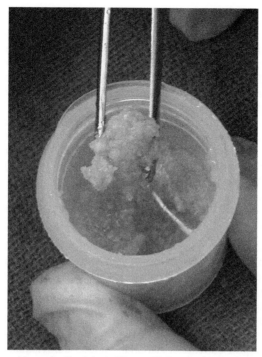

Fig. 1. Trinity is stored in a plastic vial at −70 to −80°C. It is slowly thawed to no more than 39°C in the operating room at the time of use. The material has the handling characteristics of soft cancellous bone.

MSCs have been demonstrated to show remarkable potential for healing of defects in long bones in multiple animal studies, and their use as an allograft material with intraoperative bone marrow concentration has gained increasing attention. As a practical matter, surgical use of MSCs is restrained by both the concern that without a carrier the grafted cells will not remain in the desired location and the variable quality of MSCs generated from the patient's own tissue. In particular, increasing patient age significantly affects the concentration of MSCs that can be generated from autograft concentration techniques. There is also increasing evidence that the relative "fitness" of MSCs may be reduced with age. Stolzing and colleagues[6] recently demonstrated multiple indices of aging including oxidative damage, reactive oxygen species (ROS) levels, p21, and p53 markers all increasing in older patient harvests. Other host factors, such as smoking and diabetes, also play a role. Unfortunately, it is these same factors that often place the patient into a high-risk category requiring a graft for augmentation in the first place.

THE RATIONALE BEHIND TRINITY

Trinity seeks to avoid these issues. First, the MSCs are adherent to the extracellular matrix of the cancellous material, thus providing a human allograft carrier to help ensure the cells remain in place. Second, efforts are made to take the material from younger donors; the average donor age for harvests in 2008 was 30. Assay of each preparation ensures a minimum concentration of 50,000 mesenchymal stem cells or osteoprogenitor cells per mL.[8]

SUITABLE USAGE

The appropriate indications for the use of Trinity Evolution, like other augmentation allograft products in foot and ankle surgery, remain ill defined. Classically autograft supplementation is considered in cases of substantial nonunion gaps, smokers, steroid users, and patients with chronic diseases such as diabetes. Although all methods may be said to have advantages and disadvantages, the distinction between Trinity and autograft MSC concentration techniques is most clear in the older or high-risk patient groups where native MSC concentration and activity may be suspect. In addition, the concentrations of MSCs achievable through culture expansion and concentration are substantially higher than through intraoperative centrifuge bone marrow concentration. Whether or not these theoretical advantages supply actual clinical benefit awaits carefully designed clinical trials.

PART II: BETA-TRICALCIUM PHOSPHATE/COLLAGEN WITH CONCENTRATED BONE MARROW ASPIRATE

When making a decision for bone grafting, the surgeon and patient may be unwilling to harvest bone from a second site. A bone graft substitute, such as beta-tricalcium phosphate with collagen, offers excellent biologic scaffold and dead space filler. The augmentation of this bone substitute with concentrated bone marrow aspirate potentially offers an even more attractive bone graft option.

The science of beta-tricalcium phosphate as a bone graft material dates far back in orthopedic history, when calcium phosphate (plaster of Paris) was found to be a resorbable bone graft substitute. Although various combinations of calcium and sodium phosphates have been tried, the microstructure of beta-tricalcium phosphate seems to be very close to cancellous bone. The incorporation of collagen into the beta-tricalcium phosphate binds proteins such as those within bone marrow aspirate. The collagen binds the proteins via electrostatic attraction forces.[9] Two commercial varieties of beta-tricalcium phosphate with collagen, IntegraOS (IntegraLifesciences, Inc, Plainsboro, NJ, USA) and Vitoss (Orthovita, Inc, Malvern, PA, USA), may differ in microstructure but clinically handle almost identically. Supplied in a 5-mL-long rectangular block, the materials resemble a tough Styrofoam and can be broken or cut into smaller pieces to fit small holes or gaps. Several varieties of beta tri-calcium phosphate have been produced, and definitive clinical outcome articles have yet to discern the best-performing graft in vivo. Although these materials are approved by the Food and Drug Administration (FDA) as bone graft, both manufacturers promote the use along with concentrated bone marrow aspirate.[10,11] Orthovita has also produced a next-generation Vitoss BA, which has added bioglass in an attempt to speed bone incorporation. The silicon and sodium liberated by the bioglass in theory attracts osteoblasts and thus speeds bone formation.[12]

The use of bone marrow aspirate (BMA) has markedly increased over the past several years in our institution as more information regarding the composition of the BMA has been found. The stem cells compose the primary element sought for differentiation into bone-forming cells and the iliac crest has a higher concentration of mesenchymal stem cells than the proximal tibia or the heel (Lew C. Schon, internal data at Union Memorial Hospital Orthobiologics Laboratory, 2009). Interestingly, the proximal tibia had the lowest concentration of stem cells, a worrisome issue for those still harvesting bone graft from that location. The other components of the concentrated bone marrow include a myriad of growth factors and cytokines; the qualitative and quantitative aspects of each are still being discovered. Still to be published are comparison studies of concentrated BMA (with or without carrier) to MSC preparations (such as Trinity). These MSC preparations, mixed with allograft cancellous bone, present a very attractive bone graft alternative to autograft in some patients.

SURGICAL TECHNIQUE FOR BONE MARROW ASPIRATION

The process of BMA has evolved into a simple procedure. Preoperatively, we usually wall off the pelvic area from the anterior iliac crest with an unsterile U-drape, then prep the crest at the same time as the leg and foot. We will usually block the anterior iliac crest with 5 to 10 mL of a lidocaine/bupivicaine solution, first the skin then the deep periosteum of the anterior iliac crest. In addition to pain control, this procedure helps confirm the location of the crest. The bordering of the crest with sterile towels is optional. We do take care not to drag the large drape over unprepped areas of the thigh or hip as we lay down the single-holed sterile drape from the leg cephalad toward the head. We cut a hole for the crest and use a clear adhesive drape over this hole to secure the crest for aspiration.

The aspiration begins with a simple incision using half of the #15 blade into the skin over the anterior iliac crest, a few centimeters behind the anterior superior iliac spine (ASIS). This small stab wound makes a much more cosmetic scar than the hole from the BMA trocar. The Biomet GPS (Biomet, Inc, Warsaw, IN, USA) harvesting trocar is then percutaneously advanced to the iliac crest and the width of the bone can be felt. The central aspect of the crest can then be entered by using a mallet to advance the trocar between the walls of the crest (**Fig. 2**). Once within, the simple aspiration into a 30-mL syringe, prefilled with 4 mL of ACD-A (acid citrate dextrose-anticoagulant),

A   **B**

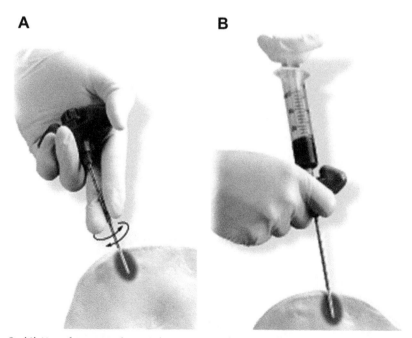

Fig. 2. (*A*) Use of trocar to harvest bone marrow between iliac walls. A mallet can also be used to advance the trocar. (*B*) Withdrawing a small amount from each segment of crest, trying to maximize bone marrow and minimize peripheral blood. (*Courtesy of* Biomet, Inc; with permission.)

yields the BMA. The choice of 30 or 60 mL of BMA depends on the volume of graft needed as well as the age and physiology of the patient. Younger, healthy patients can be expected to yield more BMA than older osteoporotic patients. Harvesting technique can vary greatly, as too much fluid aspiration at one site will begin to mix peripheral blood with bone marrow; we try to limit harvest to 10 mL from each trocar plunge.

Once collected, the BMA gets passed off to a technician who spins it down in a centrifuge with proprietary filters (Biomet GPS). This spin-down process yields 2 batches of BMA concentrate, labeled from the previous generation of peripheral blood spin-downs, PRP (platelet-rich plasma) and PPP (platelet poor plasma) (**Fig. 3**). The PRP represents the marrow stem cell–rich portion of the BMA. The block of beta-tricalcium phosphate /collagen can then be broken into several small 1- to 2-mL blocks and soaked in the PRP stem cell–rich aspirate. The smaller sizes allow for better and more rapid absorption of the aspirate into the graft. This absorption may take several minutes and thus should be performed well ahead of the timing for graft application.

The bone graft can be applied once the PRP is well absorbed; the material handles easily and compacts well into small crevices and spaces (**Figs. 4** and **5**). It has minimal strength in compression or tension and can be used to augment a corticocancellous graft (we like to burr a central groove or pack along the outside of such a graft) or cancellous chips. The product brochure for Mozaic (a different configuration of the beta-tricalcium phosphate and collagen from IntegraLifesciences) states that this configuration has much better compression resistance but these authors' experience is limited. The surgeon should take care to irrigate the surgical site before placement of the graft because the stem cell–rich iliac crest bone marrow aspirate–beta-tricalcium phosphate graft should not be diluted with saline after instillation. The graft can be mixed with allograft; some have even augmented the graft with bone morphogenic protein-2 in complex cases to promote osteogenesis. Another promotion of bone growth can be an internal or external bone stimulator, although studies of the benefits

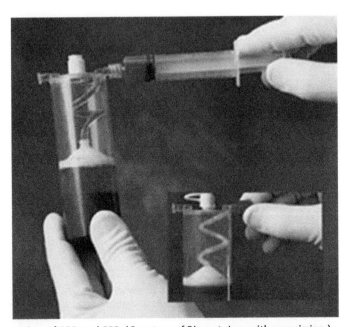

Fig. 3. Separation of PRP and PPP. (*Courtesy of* Biomet, Inc; with permission.)

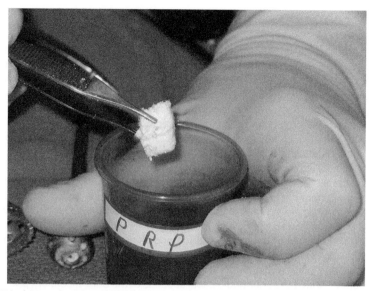

Fig. 4. Tricalcium phosphate/collagen material broken into a smaller piece.

with a bone marrow/beta-tricalcium phosphate graft have not been performed to these authors' knowledge.

The PPP component of the bone marrow aspirate has garnished an anecdotal reputation for great utility in wound healing. Several surgeons use the fluid in the subcutaneous tissues to diminish inflammation; the PPP is injected in the subcutaneous tissue after wound closure. Although no hard data have been presented, these authors have also enjoyed beneficial results over several years using this technique, described by fellow surgeon Lew C. Schon (personal communication, 2008).

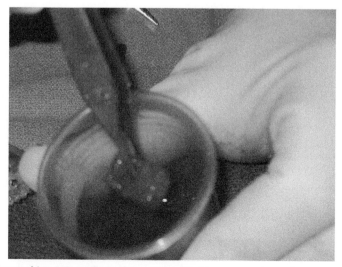

Fig. 5. After soaking IntegraOS in the concentrated bone marrow aspirate.

SUMMARY

The concept of osteoinduction and osteoconduction has been furthered with the concept of osteogenesis; Siegel and colleagues[13] discuss the scaffolding of the tricalcium phosphate/collagen for osteoconduction, the growth factors in the concentrated bone marrow aspirate for osteoinduction, and the stem cells in the concentrated bone marrow aspirate as further stimulus for osteogenesis. The scientific studies have led to various conclusions regarding the best combination of substrate and biologic agent. Castellani and colleagues[14] found no improvement in bone ingrowth between TricOs (Baxter AG, Vienna, Austria) and Collagraft (Zimmer, Inc, Warsaw, IN, USA), both tricalcium phosphates with a bioactive matrix, when bone marrow aspirate was added to the ceramics filling a rabbit femoral defect. In contrast, Liu and colleagues[15] found that human bone marrow stromal cells greatly augmented the bone formation in beta-tricalcium phosphate scaffolds when implanted into mice. Hing and colleagues[16] discussed finding in spine grafting that some of the tricalcium phosphates might be degraded early, thus decoupling bone regeneration and resorption and leading to incomplete bone repair. Their studies led to conclusion that a silicone-calcium phosphate led to a more stable osteoconductive scaffold, which thus better supported angiogenesis and bone apposition.

Recent spine work has confirmed clinical success of the beta-tricalcium phosphate/collagen combination. The beta-tricalcium phosphate has been used clinically with allograft[17] and autograft[18,19] for lumbar interbody fusion. The beta-tricalcium phosphate has been compared clinically with iliac crest autograft for posterior correction of scoliosis with equivalent fusion and less morbidity.[20] This entire issue could be devoted to comparing and contrasting the myriad of studies available; a consensus has yet to be clearly made as to the best combination of materials for bone grafting and augmentation. The authors have found great clinical success using the material in the foot and ankle, especially with concentrated bone marrow aspirate, and clinical outcome studies are under way.

REFERENCES

1. Ryan JM, Barry FP, Murphy JM, et al. Mesenchymal stem cells avoid allogeneic rejection. J Inflamm (Lond) 2005;2:8.
2. Blair HC, Zaidi M, Schlesinger PH. Mechanisms balancing skeletal matrix synthesis and degradation. Biochem J 2002;364:329–41.
3. Pittenger MF, Mackay AM, Beck SC, et al. Multilineage potential of adult human mesenchymal stem cells. Science 1999;284:143–7.
4. Hegner B, Weber M, Dragun D, et al. Differential regulation of smooth muscle markers in human bone marrow-derived mesenchymal stem cells. J Hypertens 2005;23:1191–202.
5. Jang YK, Jung DH, Jung MH, et al. Mesenchymal stem cells feeder layer from human umbilical cord blood for ex vivo expanded growth and proliferation of hematopoietic progenitor cells. Ann Hematol 2006;85:212–25.
6. Stolzing A, Jones E, McGonagle D, et al. Age-related changes in human bone marrow-derived mesenchymal stem cells: consequences for cell therapies. Mech Ageing Dev 2008;129:163–73.
7. Caplan A. Why are MSC's therapeutic? new data: new insight. J Pathol 2009;217: 318–24.
8. Musculoskeletal transplant foundation, Orthofix, Verona, Italy. "Trinity evolution" clinical data sheet 2009.
9. Mozaic product brochure. Integra life sciences, Inc, Plainsboro (NJ); 2008.

10. Vitoss product brochure. Orthovita Inc, Malvern (PA); 2009.

11. Ullrich PF. Interbody fusion using VITOSS scaffold with autogenous bone marrow aspirate—one year interim results. Orthovita, Malvern (PA): Internal White Paper Publication; 2006.

12. The use of bioactive glass in orthopaedics: improvements in healing with vitoss bioactive glass substitute, a white paper from Orthovita, Inc, Malvern (PA); 2008.

13. Siegel HJ, Baird RC, Hall J, et al. The outcome of composite bone graft substitute to treat cavitary bone defects. Orthopedics 2008;31(8):754.

14. Castellani C, Zanoni G, Tangl S, et al. Biphasic calcium phosphate ceramics in small bone defects: potential influence of carrier substances and bone marrow on bone regeneration. Clin Oral Implants Res 2009;20(12):1367–74.

15. Liu G, Zhao L, Cui L, et al. "Tissue engineered bone formation using human bone marrow stromal cells and novel beta-tricalcium phosphate". Biomed Mater. 2007; 2(2):78–86.

16. Hing KA, Wilson LF, Buckland T. Comparative performance of three ceramic bone graft substitutes. Spine J 2007;7(4):475–90.

17. Linovitz RJ, Peppers TA. Use of an advanced formulation of beta-tricalcium phosphate as a bone extender in interbody lumbar fusion. Orthopedics 2002; 25(5):S585–9.

18. Meadows GR. Adjunctive use of ultraporous beta-tricalcium phosphate void filler in spinal arthrodesis. Orthopedics 2002;25(5):s579–84.

19. Epstein NE. Non-instrumented posterolateral lumbar fusions utilizing combined lamina autograft and beta tricalcium phosphate in a predominately geriatric population: an outcome assessment. Spinal Surg 2006;20(4):219–31.

20. Lerner T, Bullmann V, Schulte TL, et al. A level-1 pilot study to evaluate ultraporous beta-tricalcium phosphate as a graft extender in the posterior correction of adolescent idiopathic scoliosis. Eur Spine J 2009;18(2):170–9.

The Evolution of rhPDGF-BB in Musculoskeletal Repair and its Role in Foot and Ankle Fusion Surgery

Christopher W. DiGiovanni, MD[a],*, James M. Petricek, MSE, MBA[b]

KEYWORDS

- Platelet-derived growth factor • Bone grafting • Arthrodesis
- Orthopedic surgery

OUR HISTORIC STANDARD: AUTOGENOUS BONE GRAFT

Arthrodesis is the standard treatment for end-stage arthritis of the foot and ankle. An estimated 110,000 arthrodesis procedures were performed in the United States in 2009.[1] A recent meta-analysis of the orthopedic literature suggests that the overall nonunion rate for ankle arthrodesis is about 10%,[2] although other studies looking at broad patient populations that include additional surgical risk factors such as a history of smoking, diabetes, avascular necrosis, or posttraumatic arthritis, have documented that the incidence of nonunion during foot and ankle fusion surgery can approach 16% to 41%.[3,4] To mitigate the risk of nonunion, autogenous bone graft is often used as an adjuvant to enhance bone healing and fill defects at the site of fusion. When arthrodesis procedures are performed around the foot and ankle, bone graft is routinely harvested from a number of anatomic sites, including the iliac crest,[5] proximal tibia,[6] distal tibia, and calcaneus.[7]

Although autogenous bone graft is probably still considered the most effective enhancer of bone healing, the incidence of complications and postoperative morbidity following bone graft harvest are well documented and have been reported to be as high as 23% in recent literature.[8] Specific donor-site complications include prolonged

[a] Division of Foot and Ankle Surgery, Department of Orthopaedic Surgery, The Warren Alpert School of Medicine at Brown University, Rhode Island Hospital, 593 Eddy Street, Providence, RI 02904, USA
[b] BioMimetic Therapeutics, Inc, 389 Nichol Mill Lane, Franklin, TN 37067, USA
* Corresponding author.
E-mail address: christopher_digiovanni@brown.edu

Foot Ankle Clin N Am 15 (2010) 621–640
doi:10.1016/j.fcl.2010.07.001
1083-7515/10/$ – see front matter © 2010 Elsevier Inc. All rights reserved.

donor-site pain,[9] infection,[10] fracture,[11] seroma formation,[12] wound complications,[8] sensory loss,[13] and scarring.[14] Of these, long-term donor site pain is perhaps the most frequently reported complication. A recently published prospective clinical study examined the effects of long-term donor site pain following iliac crest bone graft harvest on postoperative patient quality of life and function.[15] This study demonstrated that a relatively large percentage of patients (as high as 25% according to some criteria) experience significant impairment of and interference with routine activities of daily living for up to 3 years following surgery. Although this study focused on the morbidity of iliac crest graft, it is important to recognize that the postoperative pain and morbidity of bone grafting is not limited to the iliac crest. Frohberg and Mazock[16] evaluated the morbidity associated with harvesting graft from the proximal tibia. In their series, complications occurred in 19% of patients, which included prolonged donor-site pain, gait disturbances, seroma formation, paresthesia, and scarring.

In addition to patient morbidity, other limitations of autogenous bone graft include its cost and the amount of material that can be harvested. Bone grafting is frequently assumed to be a cost-effective treatment, but several studies have demonstrated that the direct and indirect costs of harvesting autogenous bone graft are substantial. Polly and colleagues[17] calculated the economic impact of harvesting iliac crest bone graft and determined that the incremental, direct medical costs average $2365 (2001 dollars) when operating room time, instrument costs, anesthesia costs, physician fees, and management of postoperative complications are considered. With respect to quantity, surgeons are continually challenged with the fact that the amount of graft that can be safely and reasonably harvested is quite finite. As an example, in a cadaveric study across multiple specimens, it was determined that an average of only 5.4 mL of compressed graft can be reasonably harvested from the proximal tibia, which arguably represents one of the most fruitful locations for bone graft regularly sought by the foot and ankle surgeon.[18] Given the various pathologies commonly affecting the foot and ankle, this amount of graft can be insufficient, depending on the size of the bone defect at the primary surgical site, the physical size of the patient, or the number of joints to be fused. Additional patient factors may also influence the amount of harvestable graft. Patients with osteoporosis, who by definition have reduced bone mineral density, may lack sufficient quantities of autogenous graft at multiple donor sites or be susceptible to fracture at the donor site. Further, patients who have had prior autograft surgery or arthroplasty may also be unable to donate graft from certain frequently used sites.

THE ADVENT OF ORTHOBIOLOGIC TECHNOLOGY

The significant limitations of the autogenous bone graft—morbidity, cost, quantity—have compelled surgeons to evaluate, and industry to develop, off-the-shelf alternatives to autogenous graft. Recombinant human platelet-derived growth factor (rhPDGF-BB), in combination with osteoconductive scaffolds, represents one of the newest orthobiologic products developed as a replacement for autogenous graft. The product (Augment Bone Graft, BioMimetic Therapeutics, Franklin, TN, USA) combines rhPDGF-BB with beta tricalcium phosphate (β-TCP) granules. Over the past several years, this combination drug/device product has been the subject of several clinical studies designed to evaluate the safety and efficacy of this material as a viable alternative to autograft in foot and ankle arthrodesis surgery. To follow is a review of the basic science and mechanism of action of PDGF in the bone-healing and regenerative process. Development of a recombinant form of PDGF, rhPDGF-BB, is also discussed, along with the history of its clinical application to date, including its current use in foot and ankle fusion procedures.

BASIC SCIENCE OF PDGF

PDGF is a naturally occurring molecule released from the α-granules of platelets, as part of the clotting process that occurs in response to injury. PDGF is both a potent mitogen and powerful chemotactic agent for cells of mesenchymal origin—including mesenchymal stem cells (MSCs), osteoblasts, fibroblasts, and vascular smooth muscle cells.[19–21] Although PDGF was first identified and isolated from platelets,[22] the name is a bit of a misnomer because it was later discovered that PDGF is expressed by a number of cell types, including megakaryocytes, macrophages, osteoblasts, and fibroblasts (**Table 1**).[23,24] The vital importance of PDGF as an early initiator of both wound healing[25] and bone regeneration[26] is well established.

Structurally, PDGF is a glycoprotein of 27,000 to 31,000 Da and is composed of 2 polypeptide chains linked by disulfide bonds.[27] Each chain is approximately 100 amino acid residues in length.[21] Within each chain, 6 cystine amino acid residues are linked together in what is termed a "cystine knot," and 2 additional cystine residues form the interchain bonds.[28] The cystine knot is a conformational feature shared by both the vascular endothelial growth factor (VEGF) family as well as placental growth factor.[21]

In reality, PDGF is a family of growth factors, which includes PDGF-A, B, C, and D. The protein, however, is biologically active only in the form of a dimer. PDGF-A and PDGF-B are capable of forming both heterodimers and homodimers, whereas PDGF-C and PDGF-D can exist only as homodimers.[26] All combinations of the PDGF molecule bind via 2 cell-surface receptors known as PDGFR-α and PDGFR-β, although PDGF-BB is the only isomer that can bind to all known PDGF receptor isotypes (**Table 2**).[21,29] Thus, PDGF-BB is considered the universal PDGF isoform, rendering it the most logical form of the protein to develop as a therapeutic.

ROLE OF PDGF IN BONE FORMATION

Bone repair is characterized by a number of distinct but overlapping stages of cellular activity. Broadly, the process begins with stabilization of a blood clot, which is

Table 1
Normal cell types expressing PDGF

Cell Type	PDGF-α Receptor	PDGF-β Receptor
Osteoblasts	+	+
Mesenchymal stem cells	+	+
Pericytes	+	+
Vascular smooth muscle cells	+	+
Platelets/megakaryocytes	+	+
Fibroblasts	+	+
Macrophages		+
Myoblasts	+	
Neurons	+	+

Abbreviation: PDGF, platelet-derived growth factor.
Data from Refs.[21,23,31,64]

Table 2
PDGF isomer/receptor binding specificity

PDGF Receptor Isotype				
		PDGFR-αα	PDGFR-αβ	PDGFR-ββ
PDGF Isomer	PDGF-AA	X		
	PDGF-AB		X	
	PDGF-BB	X	X	X
	PDGF-CC	X	X	
	PDGF-DD		X	X

PDGF-BB is the universal PDGF isomer and binds to all 3 combinations of PDGF receptors.
Abbreviation: PDGF, platelet-derived growth factor.
Data from Hollinger JO, Hart CE, Hirsch SN, et al. Recombinant human platelet-derived growth factor: biology and clinical applications. J Bone Joint Surg Am 2008;90(Suppl 1):48–54.

followed by the recruitment and proliferation of mesenchymal cells to initiate and direct repair. As the number of responding cells increases, differentiation factors activate the transformation of osteoprogenitor cells into osteoblasts, which in turn initiates the production of extracellular matrix, or "soft callus." Over time, the extracellular matrix calcifies to form woven bone, or "hard callus." In the final stage of repair, bone remodels into a lamellar structure, regaining its preinjury strength and morphology (**Fig. 1**).

PDGF is responsible for keying the early phases of the bone-healing cascade primarily through the recruitment and mitogenesis of mesenchymal stem cells (MSCs) and osteoblasts,[26] both of which are necessary to initiate bone formation (**Fig. 2**). By triggering an influx of reparative cells and causing them to divide, the dual actions of PDGF ensures a large number of appropriate cell types are available to potentiate bone repair and regeneration. The primary source of PDGF in normal bone healing is α-granule degranulation from platelets activated by a paracrine signaling mechanism. PDGF can also be expressed, however, through an autocrine signaling pathway, via cells recruited by PDGF such as macrophages and osteoblasts. This observation was first made by Fujii and colleagues,[24] and later demonstrated

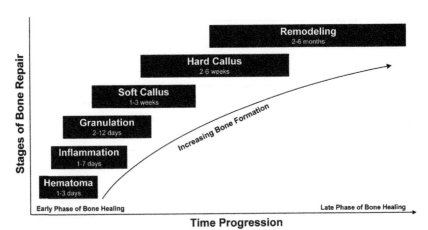

Fig. 1. Overview of bone repair process. (*Data from* Refs.[26,62,63])

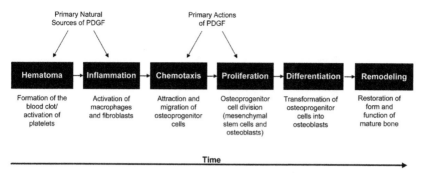

Fig. 2. The role of PDGF in bone formation. The expression and activity of PDGF occurs early in the bone-repair cascade by attracting and proliferating the appropriate cell types to potentiate bone regeneration.

through a series of experiments by Huang and colleagues[30] in a model of normal bone formation. In these studies, the expression of PDGF mRNA expression was measured longitudinally at several time points (**Fig. 3**). The results demonstrated a bimodal release pattern, suggesting multiple cell sources for PDGF. Also notable from these data is the expression of PDGF relative to the expression of BMP (**Fig. 4**). Maximal expression of PDGF is distinct from BMP, and occurs upstream (ie, earlier) in the bone repair cascade.

PDGF MECHANISM OF ACTION

The ability to simultaneously influence cellular chemotaxis, mitogenesis, and angiogenesis is what distinguishes PDGF from other therapeutic proteins.

Chemotaxis

Chemotaxis is a phenomenon whereby cells physically migrate in response to a stimulus. A number of growth proteins involved with bone repair have been shown to

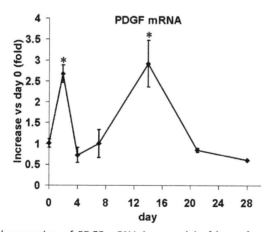

Fig. 3. Sequential expression of PDGF mRNA in a model of bone formation. *, Indicates statistical significance (*P*<.05) relative to day 0; #, indicates statistical significance relative to days 0 and 2. (*From* Huang Z, Nelson ER, Smith RL, et al. The sequential expression profiles of growth factors from osteoprogenitors to osteoblasts in vitro. Tissue Eng 2007;13(9): 2311–20; with permission.)

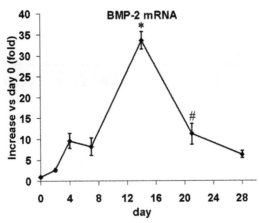

Fig. 4. Sequential expression of BMP mRNA in a model of bone formation. As shown in a model of normal, healthy bone repair, PDGF is naturally expressed bimodally, both early (within 2 days of injury) in the healing cascade as well as at 2 weeks, whereas the expression of BMP occurs primarily later (at 2 weeks) in the reparative sequence. These data compare the levels of protein to baseline. *, Indicates statistical significance (P<.05) relative to day 0; #, indicates statistical significance relative to days 0 and 2. (*From* Huang Z, Nelson ER, Smith RL, et al. The sequential expression profiles of growth factors from osteoprogenitors to osteoblasts in vitro. Tissue Eng 2007;13(9):2311–20; with permission.)

possess chemotactic activity toward mesenchymal stem cells, including transforming growth factor (TGF), fibroblast growth factor (FGF), insulin-like growth factor (IGF), and thrombin.[19] The chemotactic potency toward mesenchymal stem cells, however, differs markedly between proteins. In numerous experiments, PDGF has been shown to be the most potent chemotactic agent for mesenchymal stem cells.[19,31,32] Fiedler and colleagues[32] demonstrated the superior chemotactic activity of PDGF in comparison with BMP-2, BMP-4, TGF-β, and FGF (**Fig. 5**).

Mitogenesis

Mitogenesis is a phenomenon whereby cells divide (proliferate) in response to a stimulus. PDGF is also a powerful mitogen for all cells of mesenchymal origin. As part of the original research that led to the discovery of PDGF,[22] it was observed that exposure of cells to blood serum (containing platelets) promoted the proliferation of cells in culture. Since these early investigations, the mitogenic capacity of PDGF toward mesenchymal stem cells has been compared with other common bone proteins. In studies conducted by Ozaki and colleagues,[19] a radiolabeled [³H] thymidine assay was used to assess the mitogenic capacity of PDGF (AA, AB, BB) relative to 20 other growth proteins and cytokines. The results from this investigation illustrate the dramatic influence of PDGF on the replication of mesenchymal stem cells relative to BMP-2 and the other growth factors and cytokines tested (**Fig. 6**).

Angiogenesis

Without exception, successful bone healing and regeneration is dependent upon access to a viable blood supply. Sufficient blood flow is required to deliver nutrients and oxygen, permit ingress of bone-forming cells, and facilitate egress of cellular debris and other waste products. PDGF, in addition to its significant role in stimulating the recruitment and proliferation of bone-forming cells, has been shown to

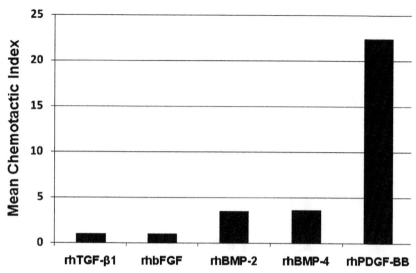

Fig. 5. Chemotactic potential of PDGF for human mesenchymal progenitor cells. Human mesenchymal stem cells were obtained from consented donors and evaluated for chemotactic response using a modified Boyden chamber assay, a common technique used to measure cellular migration. The cells were separately exposed to several bone proteins at various concentrations and tested in triplicate. The diagram compares the chemotactic response of the cells when exposed to 1 ng/mL of each respective protein. Results are expressed in units of chemotactic index (CI), which is the ratio of the number of cells that migrate in response to exposure to a stimulus as compared with controls. rhPDGF-BB was the most potent chemokine tested. (*Data from* Fiedler J, Röderer G, Günther KP, et al. BMP-2, BMP-4, and PDGF-BB stimulate chemotactic migration of primary human mesenchymal progenitor cells. J Cell Biochem 2002;87(3):305–12.)

increase angiogenesis both directly and through up-regulating the expression of the pro-angiogenic molecule vascular endothelial growth factor (VEGF) from osteoblasts in a dose-dependent manner (**Fig. 7**).[33] Further, this angiogenic effect is enhanced in the presence of hypoxia, which is a characteristic of the fracture microenvironment.

PDGF receptors (α and β) are also expressed on pericytes (ie, mural cells), a type of perivascular endothelial cell that envelops the outer surface of capillaries.[21,34] This is significant because it demonstrates that PDGF not only encourages neoangiogenesis by up-regulating the expression of VEGF, but also recruits and expands the number of pericytes, which are needed to stabilize and strengthen the newly formed blood vessels.

DEVELOPMENT OF rhPDGF-BB AS A THERAPEUTIC: HUMAN STUDIES

With the basic science of endogenous PDGF as a backdrop, significant interest began to heighten in the 1980s to develop a recombinant human form of PDGF for therapeutic use. During that period, methods to produce recombinant human PDGF (rhPDGF-BB, INN: becaplermin) in a yeast expression system were established, hence creating the means to develop commercial therapies with the molecule.

Among other strategies to produce rhPDGF-BB, the human gene that encodes the amino acid sequence of the PDGF-B chain was introduced into *Saccharomyces cerevisiae* cells (ie, Brewer's/Baker's yeast). During yeast fermentation, the gene is expressed, leading to the synthesis of the PDGF-B chain polypeptide. Within the

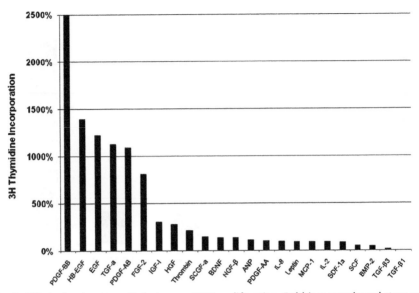

Fig. 6. Effect of various growth factors on MSC proliferation. Rabbit mesenchymal stem cells (MSC) were separately exposed to 23 different growth factors and cytokines in an ^{3}H thymidine assay, which is commonly used to assess cell proliferation. In this assay, the uptake of thymidine is proportional to the level of cell proliferation. The experiment was run in triplicate; average values are reported. Values are expressed as a percentage of control. rhPDGF-BB was the most potent growth factor tested. (*Data from* Ozaki Y, Nishimura M, Sekiya K, et al. Comprehensive analysis of chemotactic factors for bone marrow mesenchymal stem cells. Stem Cells Dev 2007;16(1):119–29.)

cell, the chains undergo cross-linking and fold into a 3-dimensional conformation to form the BB dimer. The cross-linked protein is subsequently secreted from the yeast cell into the culture medium and purified through a multistep process. Currently, all rhPDGF-BB intended for human use is produced via this yeast expression system in a good manufacturing practice (GMP)-compliant manufacturing facility (Novartis, Emeryville, CA, USA) approved by the Food and Drug Administration (FDA).

The development of recombinant human PDGF (rhPDGF-BB) for commercial purposes was initially focused on soft tissue wound healing through the development of Regranex (Systagenix Wound Management, Quincy, MA, USA), and later concentrated on regeneration of periodontal bone loss through the development of GEM 21S (BioMimetic Therapeutics, Franklin, TN, USA and Osteohealth Co, Shirley, NY, USA).

Regranex

Regranex (0.01% rhPDGF-BB) gel was developed as a topical ointment for the treatment of lower extremity diabetic neuropathic ulcers. In 1997, this product received FDA approval on the basis of the clinical results from 4 multicenter, randomized, placebo-controlled trials. In these studies, which encompassed a total of 922 subjects, patients treated with Regranex gel in combination with good ulcer care (defined as sharp debridement before randomization and regular dressing changes) demonstrated consistently higher levels of complete ulcer healing in comparison with patients treated with good ulcer care alone.[35] In a subsequent retrospective

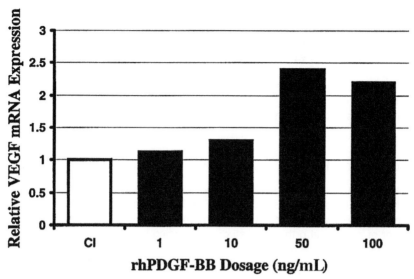

Fig. 7. Expression of VEGF mRNA from osteoblasts in response to PDGF exposure. Rat calvarial osteoblast cell cultures were separately exposed to various doses of rhPDGF-BB. Subsequent VEGF mRNA expression was evaluated using Northern blot analysis. The experiment was run in duplicate. These data demonstrate that rhPDGF-BB enhances the expression of VEGF mRNA in a dose-dependent manner. (*From* Bouletreau PJ, Warren SM, Spector JA, et al. Factors in the fracture microenvironment induce primary osteoblast angiogenic cytokine production. Plast Reconstr Surg 2002;110(1):139–48; with permission.)

study, 22,504 patients treated for diabetic neuropathic foot ulcers were compared with 2394 treated for the same condition with Regranex gel.[36] In this larger study, wounds treated with Regranex demonstrated a 32% higher likelihood to heal in comparison with controls.

GEM 21S

GEM 21S (0.3 mg/mL rhPDGF-BB/β-TCP granules) was subsequently developed as a grafting material to fill and regenerate bony defects as a consequence of advanced periodontal disease. The product received FDA approval in 2005 on the basis of a multicenter, prospective, blinded, randomized, and controlled clinical trial to evaluate the product's safety and efficacy in this indication. The clinical trial encompassed 180 subjects enrolled at 11 institutions, with each patient having a least one osseous defect greater than 4 mm in depth. The study was randomized 1:1:1 such that equal numbers of subjects received β-TCP alone or β-TCP in combination with 1 of 2 doses of rhPDGF-BB (0.3 mg/mL or 1.0 mg/mL). Patients treated with rhPDGF-BB demonstrated statistically significant increases in clinical attachment level (CAL) at 3 months and significantly greater radiographic linear bone growth and percentage bone fill at 6 months as compared with patients treated with β-TCP alone.[37] Further, no significant device-related adverse events were observed in patients receiving the rhPDGF-BB treatment. In this study, patients treated with the 0.3 mg/mL concentration of rhPDGF-BB demonstrated the best overall clinical outcomes, which represents the rationale for using the 0.3 mg/mL dose in all subsequent clinical studies in orthopedics. Several postmarketing clinical trials also have been published in periodontal and oral and maxillofacial reconstructive indications including alveolar ridge reconstruction, maxillary sinus floor augmentation, tooth extraction sockets, and gingival recession. These trials have demonstrated the safety and effectiveness of rhPDGF-BB in combination with various matrices preferred by the clinicians, including bone allograft and autograft/allograft mixtures for osseous reconstruction and collagen meshes for periodontal ligament and other soft tissue reconstruction indications.[38–42] It is estimated that more than 100,000 patients were treated with rhPDGF-BB in orofacial indications between January 2006 and January 2010.

DEVELOPMENT OF rhPDGF-BB AS A THERAPEUTIC: ANIMAL RESEARCH

The clinical and commercial success of both Regranex and GEM 21S have most recently led to the development of rhPDGF-BB for orthopedic applications. To this end, rhPDGF-BB, in combination with a matrix or scaffold, has been evaluated in a number of preclinical orthopedic studies, including geriatric osteoporotic fracture repair,[43] diabetic fracture repair,[44] and distraction osteogenesis.[45]

In the osteoporotic fracture study, geriatric rats with low bone mass were treated with 1 of 2 doses of rhPDGF-BB (0.3 mg/mL or 1.0 mg/mL) in combination with a β-TCP and collagen matrix in a model of tibial fracture repair.[43] At 3 and 5 weeks postoperative, both rhPDGF-BB groups exhibited moderate to marked bridging callus across the fracture site, whereas nontreated and matrix-alone treated (no rhPDGF-BB) animals exhibited minimal bone healing with little to no callus formation. Also at 5 weeks, improved biomechanical properties (torque to failure) were demonstrated in the fractured tibiae treated with rhPDGF-BB/collagen/TCP compared with the control groups.

In the diabetic fracture repair study, diabetic BB Wistar rats with middiaphyseal femur fractures were treated with (1) rhPDGF-BB/collagen/β-TCP, (2) matrix alone (no rhPDGF), or (3) no treatment.[44] rhPDGF-BB–treated animals exhibited significantly higher levels of callus cellular proliferation early (4 days after fracture). This also translated into improved biomechanical and histologic properties at later time points (8 and 12 weeks after fracture) as compared with the control animals.

In a model of distraction osteogenesis, rhPDGF-BB in combination with a soluble collagen matrix was locally injected weekly into the femoral distraction site of a rat over a 4-week period, coinciding with the time frame of mechanical distraction.[45] Bone healing was analyzed through serial radiographs, postmortem micro CT, and histomorphometric analysis of the explanted bones. Serial radiographs demonstrated statistically significantly higher levels of new bone formation in rhPDGF-BB–treated animals that were humanely killed 2, 3, or 4 weeks after the distraction period as compared with controls. Micro CT and histologic analyses confirmed these results, and consistently demonstrated higher levels of new bone formation in rhPDGF-BB–treated animals as compared with controls.

Collectively, these studies demonstrated the positive effect of local application of rhPDGF-BB on bone formation, and provided additional scientific rationale to clinically evaluate Augment Bone Graft (0.3 mg/mL rhPDGF-BB/β-TCP granules) as a purely synthetic replacement to autograft in hindfoot and ankle arthrodesis surgery. Augment is similar in design to GEM 21S, but is offered in larger quantities, greater particle sizes (β-TCP granules), and sterile packaging to account for the differences in treatment paradigms between these two applications. Foot and ankle arthrodesis was selected as a representative and challenging indication to clinically evaluate this product's safety and efficacy in an orthopedic setting. Several prospective clinical trials have been conducted and others are in progress to determine the safety and efficacy of Augment in foot and ankle arthrodesis.

AUGMENT BONE GRAFT IN FOOT AND ANKLE ARTHRODESIS
Prospective 60-Patient Open-Label Canadian Registration Trial

This study was a prospective, open-label, multicenter trial designed to evaluate Augment Bone Graft in patients requiring ankle, hindfoot, or midfoot arthrodesis. Sixty patients were enrolled across 3 institutions following approval of the clinical trial protocol by the local Research Ethics Boards (REB) and Health Canada. All patients received Augment Bone Graft in lieu of autogenous bone graft to facilitate bony healing, and were followed for 36 weeks. Patients received regular clinical and radiographic review postoperatively. CT scans of the fusion site were also obtained at 6 and 12 weeks, with an optional CT scan provided at 16 weeks.

All surgeries for these clinical studies were performed by orthopedic surgeons who were members of the American and/or Canadian Orthopaedic Foot and Ankle Societies and fellowship-trained in foot and ankle reconstruction. The surgical techniques involving joint exposure, debridement of articular cartilage, and perforation of the articular surfaces were standardized. Rigid fixation of the joint was accomplished through the use of screws (3.5 to 7.3 mm, depending on the size of the patient's foot). No more than 4 screws were used across a given fusion space to ensure adequate visualization during follow-up imaging. Plate fixation was expressly excluded owing to both the potential for radiographic scatter on CT scans as well as the intent to standardize the fixation hardware. Augment Bone Graft was packed into the fusion site at the time of rigid fixation, such that the graft material was in contact with a large amount of surface area of both bone ends, but did not cause any distraction of the joint space or in any way prevent direct coaptation of the joint surface(s). The amount of implanted material was at the surgeon's discretion, based on the number of joints to be fused and the surface area of the joint, but in no case could exceed 9 mL of total graft volume. The use of autogenous bone graft was not permitted. Layered closure was performed before deflating the tourniquet to optimize containment of the graft material within the fusion site. Postoperative care regarding short-term immobilization and weight-bearing progression was also standardized among patients. Patients transitioned to a regular walking shoe between 8 and 12 weeks. The primary efficacy end point was radiographic union, as determined by an independent radiologist assessing plain-film radiographs and CT scans. Union was declared by plain-film radiographic analysis if bridging and/or disappearance of the joint space (on at least 2 of the 4 radiologic aspects) was detected.

Of the 60 enrolled patients, 59 completed the study. Thirty-seven patients (62%) participating in the study had at least one risk factor for nonunion, including recent smoking history, diabetes, and revision surgery. By 36 weeks, 52 (88%) of 59 patients exhibited radiographic union on plain films as the primary study end point; 43% (22/51) of patients exhibited 50% or greater osseous bridging across the surface area of the joint based on 6-week CT scan assessment, using a threshold for fusion similar to that proposed by Coughlin and colleagues.[46] By the 12- to 16-week time period, 75% of patients exhibited 50% or greater osseous bridging on CT scan. Of the 60 treated patients, 54 (90%) were considered a clinical success, which meant that subjects neither required nor were recommended for revision surgery within 12 months of the index procedure (**Table 3**). Six patients (10%) in the study were determined to be clinical failures, and required or were recommended for revision surgery within 12 months of the index surgery. Five of these 6 patients, interestingly, had their

Table 3
Prospective 60-patient open-label Canadian registration trial—clinical results

End Point	Investigational Group (rhPDGF-BB/β-TCP) N = 60
CT scan (≥50% osseous bridging)	
Week 6	22/51 (43%)
Week 12	44/59 (75%)
Plain radiograph (2 of 4 aspects)	
Week 24	46/54 (85%)
Week 36	52/59 (88%)
Clinical success[a]	
Week 36	54/60 (90%)

Abbreviations: rhPDGF-BB, recombinant human platelet-derived growth factor–BB; β-TCP, beta tricalcium phosphate.
[a] Defined by subjects who were not recommended for revision surgery within 12 months of the index procedure.

procedure performed on a midfoot joint. Although the rates of radiographic nonunion observed in this study were consistent with those observed in the literature,[2,3] the results did illuminate some of the difficulties associated with midfoot fusion. It was the investigators' opinion that perhaps the use of only screws (no plates) in the midfoot potentially led to micromotion across these joints, which might have contributed to some of the nonunions, but this remains undetermined. No device-related serious adverse events were reported.

Overall, this open-label study demonstrated acceptable safety and effectiveness of Augment Bone Graft as an alternative to autogenous bone graft in foot and ankle fusion procedures, without the associated harvest site morbidity. As appropriate for a first-in-humans trial for a new indication, the primary goal of the study was to determine safety and clinical utility. As such, the investigation maximized the number of patients treated with Augment and relied on historical controls, although this could be considered a potential weakness of the investigation. Nonetheless, the study demonstrated that rhPDGF-BB combined with β-TCP led to clinical and radiologic fusion rates comparable with those reported in the literature for autogenous bone graft, and such historical control comparisons are common in the foot and ankle literature.[47]

Prospective Randomized Controlled 20-Patient US Pilot Trial

In this study, 20 adult subjects requiring ankle or hindfoot fusion from 3 US centers were consecutively enrolled and randomized 2:1 to receive Augment Bone Graft or autogenous bone graft, respectively.[48] The investigation was conducted under an FDA-approved Investigational Device Exemption (IDE). Institutional review board approval and informed consent were obtained before patient enrollment. Inclusion and exclusion criteria were strict.

Similar to the 60-patient Canadian Registration Trial described previously, the surgical approach was standardized for each hindfoot and ankle fusion procedure across all treatment centers. Before applying rigid fixation, either Augment Bone Graft or surgically harvested autogenous bone was packed into the fusion site such that graft material was in contact with the entire perimeter of the joint to be fused, but not placed in a manner that precluded direct host bone-bone apposition. Autogenous bone graft was harvested from the iliac crest, Gerdy tubercle, distal tibia, or calcaneus, per investigator preference. Following reduction and fixation, any additional residual graft material was placed around the fusion site(s) as necessary to fill any exposed voids or interstices, although limits were placed on absolute graft quantity depending on the number of joints to be fused. Closure was then meticulously performed to maximize graft containment.

Postoperatively, patients remained non–weight bearing in a cast until the week 6 visit, at which time they were advanced to a walking boot and permitted limited weight bearing. Physical therapy was then initiated and patients were progressively advanced in their weight-bearing status. All enrolled patients were followed for 36 weeks postoperatively.

The primary end point of the study was time to osseous union, as determined by plain-film radiography interpreted by a blinded independent radiologist. Radiographic union was stringently defined as osseous bridging across the subchondral surfaces of at least 3 of the 4 regions delineating each fused joint—specifically, the anterior/superior, posterior/inferior, medial, and lateral quadrants. Osseous bridging was defined as trabecular bridging across the former joint space equaling that of adjacent subchondral trabeculation and associated with complete loss of distinctiveness of bone graft particles and particle density. Interval CT scan assessments were also used in these patients to assess union, which was declared only if 50% or greater of the intended fusion site was bridged.

Radiographic union rates were similar between groups. By week 12, 41.7% (5/12) of patients in the Augment group and 33.3% (1/3) of patients who received autogenous bone graft had achieved osseous union. At week 36, 71.4% (10/14) of patients in the Augment Bone Graft group and 75.0% (3/4) of patients in the autogenous bone graft group were considered fused using the primary end point criterion. CT examination at week 6 demonstrated union in 38.5% (5/13) of the Augment Bone Graft patients versus 40.0% (2/5) of the autogenous bone graft patients, and by week 12 these numbers were, respectively, 69.2% (9/13) versus 60.0% (3/5) (**Table 4**). In cases

Table 4
Prospective randomized controlled 20-patient US pilot trial—clinical results

End Point	Investigational Group (rhPDGF-BB/β-TCP) N = 14	Control Group (Autograft) N = 6
CT scan (≥50% osseous bridging)		
Week 6	5/13 (38%)	2/5 (40%)
Week 12	9/13 (69%)	3/5 (60%)
Plain radiograph (3 of 4 aspects)		
Week 12	5/12 (42%)	1/3 (33%)
Week 36	10/14 (71%)	3/4 (75%)
Clinical success[a]		
Week 36	11/13 (85%)	6/6 (100%)

Abbreviations: rhPDGF-BB, recombinant human platelet-derived growth factor–BB; β-TCP, beta tricalcium phosphate.
[a] Defined by subjects who were not recommended for revision surgery within 12 months of the index procedure.

where films were uninterpretable or missing, fusion success was not determined at that time point.

At final follow-up (36 weeks), the overall clinical success rate was 85% for the Augment group and 100% for the autogenous bone graft group. In terms of functional outcome, physician- and patient-scored American Orthopaedic Foot and Ankle Society (AOFAS) Ankle-Hindfoot Scale numbers were comparable between the Augment and autogenous bone graft groups (56.2 vs 54.8) at 12 weeks respectively, although at 36 weeks a difference was noted between the groups (71.1 vs 82.2). Two nonunions occurred in the Augment group that required reoperation, and both were thought by the investigators to be primarily responsible for the observed final differences between clinical success and functional outcomes scores. Both patients were revised using autogenous bone graft, and one of these revisions also failed to unite after this additional surgery. Upon review of both delayed/nonunions in this study, the treating surgeons felt that there had been an excessive volume of β-TCP implanted between the joint spaces intended for fusion—which may have acted as a mechanical distractor of the joint. Based on this early observation, greater attention was subsequently paid to the technique in successive patients to avoid what was considered a technical error impeding primary host bone-bone apposition.

Despite these challenges, this study illuminated a number of positives. Most importantly, there were no serious device-related adverse events observed in this study. Additionally, patients who received Augment Bone Graft were spared the pain associated with autograft harvest, which was significant in this series (mean postoperative donor site Visual Analog Scale score was 45.3) among autograft patients, who continued to report donor site pain at 36 weeks. Further, operating room time was reduced by an average of 26 minutes when Augment Bone Graft was used in place of autograft during the procedure(s).

The promising results from this prospective, randomized, controlled feasibility study, although encompassing a smaller number of patients relative to the Canadian study, established additional safety and efficacy data for Augment Bone Graft. The experience from this trial provided the impetus for designing and initiating a larger, statistically powered, pivotal clinical trial to more completely and scientifically assess the potential of Augment Bone Graft to replace autogenous bone graft in foot and ankle arthrodesis, as discussed in the next section.

Prospective 434-Patient North American Pivotal Trial

Most recently, Augment Bone Graft was evaluated in a large, prospective, multicenter, randomized, controlled trial across North America to definitively establish the safety and efficacy of the product as an alternative to autogenous bone graft in hindfoot and ankle arthrodesis. The trial was conducted at 37 clinical centers in the United States and Canada, and enrolled 434 patients. This study represents a major collective effort on behalf of AOFAS, and, to date, is the largest and most comprehensive study ever conducted in the subspecialty of foot and ankle surgery. Similar to the US pilot trial, the study was also randomized 2:1 to receive Augment Bone Graft versus autogenous bone graft. Strict enrollment criteria were maintained in accordance with prior studies, and both the surgical and postoperative treatments were similarly standardized between groups. The study was powered for statistical noninferiority. Based on observations from the pilot study regarding the poor reliability of plain film for assessing union, the primary end point of fusion was assessed using CT scans, based on the criterion of 50% or greater osseous bridging at 24 weeks.

This trial has now been completed through 24 weeks (the primary end point) on all patients, and safety data are currently being collected and analyzed through 52 weeks postoperative. Results from this study at the 24-week end point have recently been presented, and demonstrated comparable radiographic fusion rates as well as clinical and functional outcomes between the 2 study groups, including surgeon-based, patient-based, and independent blinded radiologist-based assessment parameters.[49] These data will not be elaborated further herein, however, because a complete presentation and comprehensive assessment of the full term results of this trial are currently in preparation for publication in a major peer-reviewed journal.

DISCUSSION

As the practicing orthopedic surgeon is well aware today, there are currently a multitude of bone graft substitutes and materials that are marketed for commercial use (more than 200 products 510k cleared by FDA) with little or no supporting Level I or II clinical data. Many bone graft substitutes, including demineralized bone matrix and synthetics such as calcium phosphate and calcium sulfate, are specifically labeled as bone void fillers, for example, and are not designated as true replacements for autogenous bone graft. Neither these materials nor any cell-based technologies have been subjected to the rigors of a head-to-head comparison to autograft in a large-scale clinical foot and ankle trial to assess their safety and efficacy.

Currently, the only bone-grafting products that have been tested in rigorous, prospective, randomized controlled clinical trials are the bone morphogenic proteins rhBMP-7 (OP-1, Stryker Biotech, Hopkinton, MA, USA) and rhBMP-2 (INFUSE, Medtronic Spinal and Biologics, Memphis, TN, USA). In particular, these have been studied in alternative clinical indications such as long bone (tibial) nonunion, acute tibial fracture, and lumbar spinal fusion. OP-1 has received a very limited regulatory approval in the United States under a Humanitarian Device Exemption (HDE) but has never received a full FDA approval under the less restrictive pre-market approval, which would permit broader surgeon use. The restricted approval in the case of OP-1 is presumably the result, in part, of the failure of this particular product to meet its clinical study end points in 2 large-scale randomized controlled trials.[50,51] rhBMP-2 has shown promise as a replacement for autogenous bone, particularly in the spine literature, and there is no doubt that it is a powerful bone-forming protein and a useful adjunct to the surgeon's armamentarium. However, it is not without its own subset of limitations and risks, particularly those related to its poorer safety profile when used outside its narrowly approved label. For example, application of rhBMP-2 in the cervical spine has been associated with severe perioperative complications, including severe swelling, dysphagia, and airway compromise leading to emergent surgery and death.[52] Additionally, the use of rhBMP-2 has been associated with a number of other complications, including ectopic bone formation, when used outside the scope of its approved labeling.[53–59]

The limitations of existing bone grafting products in terms of safety, efficacy, and approved indications underscore the need for further research to improve our surgical options and provide better alternatives. The early results for Augment Bone Graft hold promise as a potential alternative solution for some of these significant shortcomings. To date, the product has been evaluated in 3 multicenter trials to evaluate its effectiveness in foot and ankle fusion surgery. In each of these investigations, the clinical safety and efficacy results have been remarkably consistent. From a safety standpoint, these trials have not resulted in any serious device-related adverse events, significant immunologic sequelae, or any other negative reactions clearly attributable to the product. With respect to efficacy, Augment Bone Graft appears to be equally efficacious in stimulating bone healing as compared with autogenous bone graft, while sparing patients the prolonged pain and morbidity that can be associated with bone harvest procedures. The platform technology in rhPDGF-BB as a product has a long clinical and commercial history (Regranex, GEM 21S), which itself is based on the comprehensive understanding of its role in regulating the wound-healing and bone-regeneration cascades.

In contradistinction to many of the other bone-grafting products currently on the market, Augment Bone Graft is undergoing rigorous evaluation through a sequential series of progressively more stringently designed and statistically powered Level I and II studies. If approved, Augment Bone Graft would thereafter represent the only recombinant therapeutic protein cleared by the FDA for use in the foot and ankle as a replacement for autogenous bone graft.

Given the fundamental role of PDGF in musculoskeletal repair and regeneration, the future role for rhPDGF-BB in orthopedic surgery is expected to expand well beyond foot and ankle fusion. Additional research is under way to further our understanding of the potential for this molecule in other bone-healing applications, as well as in indications requiring healing of tendons, ligaments, and cartilage. For example, recently presented results from studies in large animals suggest that rhPDGF-BB in combination with a collagen matrix may be useful in stimulating the healing of Achilles tendon ruptures and rotator cuff tears.[60,61] These preliminary observations, taken together with the safety and efficacy data from the large-scale foot and ankle clinical trials described previously, collectively suggest that rhPDGF-BB may be a beneficial adjunct to improving musculoskeletal tissue repair. Future investigations with rhPDGF-BB will hopefully continue to shed more light on how we can best use this molecule to further improve the outcomes of our musculoskeletal patients.

REFERENCES

1. Extremity reconstruction. Available at: http://www.pearldiverinc.com/. Accessed February 24, 2010.
2. Haddad SL, Coetzee JC, Estok R, et al. Intermediate and long-term outcomes of total ankle arthroplasty and ankle arthrodesis. A systematic review of the literature. J Bone Joint Surg Am 2007;89(9):1899–905.
3. Easley ME, Trnka HJ, Schon LC, et al. Isolated subtalar arthrodesis. J Bone Joint Surg Am 2000;82(5):613–24.
4. Frey C, Halikus NM, Vu-Rose T, et al. A review of ankle arthrodesis: predisposing factors to nonunion. Foot Ankle Int 1994;15(11):581–4.
5. DeOrio JK, Farber DC. Morbidity associated with anterior iliac crest bone grafting in foot and ankle surgery. Foot Ankle Int 2005;26(2):147–51.
6. Soohoo NF, Cracchiolo A. The results of utilizing proximal tibial bone graft in reconstructive procedures of the foot and ankle. Foot Ankle Surg 2008;14(2):62–6.
7. Raikin SM, Brislin K. Local bone graft harvested from the distal tibia or calcaneus for surgery of the foot and ankle. Foot Ankle Int 2005;26(6):449–53.
8. Ahlmann E, Patzakis M, Roidis N, et al. Comparison of anterior and posterior iliac crest bone grafts in terms of harvest-site morbidity and functional outcomes. J Bone Joint Surg Am 2002;84(5):716–20.
9. Kim DH, Rhim R, Li L, et al. Prospective study of iliac crest bone graft harvest site pain and morbidity. Spine J 2009;9(11):886–92.
10. Robertson PA, Wray AC. Natural history of posterior iliac crest bone graft donation for spinal surgery: a prospective analysis of morbidity. Spine (Phila Pa 1976) 2001; 26(13):1473–6.

11. Chou LB, Mann RA, Coughlin MJ, et al. Stress fracture as a complication of autogenous bone graft harvest from the distal tibia. Foot Ankle Int 2007;28(2): 199–201.
12. Banwart JC, Asher MA, Hassanein RS. Iliac crest bone graft harvest donor site morbidity. A statistical evaluation. Spine (Phila Pa 1976) 1995;20(9): 1055–60.
13. Kirmeier R, Payer M, Lorenzoni M, et al. Harvesting of cancellous bone from the proximal tibia under local anesthesia: donor site morbidity and patient experience. J Oral Maxillofac Surg 2007;65(11):2235–41.
14. Chen YC, Chen CH, Chen PL, et al. Donor site morbidity after harvesting of proximal tibia bone. Head Neck 2006;28(6):496–500.
15. Schwartz CE, Martha JF, Kowalski P, et al. Prospective evaluation of chronic pain associated with posterior autologous iliac crest bone graft harvest and its effect on postoperative outcome. Health Qual Life Outcomes 2009;7:49.
16. Frohberg U, Mazock JB. A review of morbidity associated with bone harvest from the proximal tibial metaphysic. Mund Kiefer Gesichtschir 2005;9(2): 63–5.
17. Polly DW Jr, Ackerman SJ, Shaffrey CI, et al. A cost analysis of bone morphogenetic protein versus autogenous iliac crest bone graft in single-level anterior lumbar fusion. Orthopedics 2003;26(10):1027–37.
18. Alt V, Meeder PJ, Seligson D, et al. The proximal tibia metaphysis: a reliable donor site for bone grafting? Clin Orthop Relat Res 2003;414:315–21.
19. Ozaki Y, Nishimura M, Sekiya K, et al. Comprehensive analysis of chemotactic factors for bone marrow mesenchymal stem cells. Stem Cells Dev 2007;16(1): 119–29.
20. Fiedler J, Etzel N, Brenner RE. To go or not to go: migration of human mesenchymal progenitor cells stimulated by isoforms of PDGF. J Cell Biochem 2004; 93(5):990–8.
21. Alvarez RH, Kantarjian HM, Cortes JE. Biology of platelet-derived growth factor and its involvement in disease. Mayo Clin Proc 2006;81(9):1241–57.
22. Ross R, Glomset J, Kariya B, et al. A platelet-dependent serum factor that stimulates the proliferation of arterial smooth muscle cells in vitro. Proc Natl Acad Sci U S A 1974;71(4):1207–10.
23. Heldin CH, Westermark B. Mechanism of action and in vivo role of platelet-derived growth factor. Physiol Rev 1999;79(4):1283–316.
24. Fujii H, Kitazawa R, Maeda S, et al. Expression of platelet-derived growth factor proteins and their receptor alpha and beta mRNAs during fracture healing in the normal mouse. Histochem Cell Biol 1999;112(2):131–8.
25. Lynch SE, Nixon JC, Colvin RB, et al. Role of platelet-derived growth factor in wound healing: synergistic effects with other growth factors. Proc Natl Acad Sci U S A 1987;84(21):7696–700.
26. Hollinger JO, Hart CE, Hirsch SN, et al. Recombinant human platelet-derived growth factor: biology and clinical applications. J Bone Joint Surg Am 2008; 90(Suppl 1):48–54.
27. Bowen-Pope DF, Malpass TW, Foster DM, et al. Platelet-derived growth factor in vivo: levels, activity, and rate of clearance. Blood 1984;64(2):458–69.
28. Sun PD, Davies DR. The cystine-knot growth-factor superfamily. Annu Rev Biophys Biomol Struct 1995;24:269–91.
29. Seifert RA, Hart CE, Phillips PE, et al. Two different subunits associate to create isoform-specific platelet-derived growth factor receptors. J Biol Chem 1989; 264(15):8771–8.

30. Huang Z, Nelson ER, Smith RL, et al. The sequential expression profiles of growth factors from osteoprogenitors to osteoblasts in vitro. Tissue Eng 2007;13(9): 2311–20.

31. Ponte AL, Marais E, Gallay N, et al. The in vitro migration capacity of human bone marrow mesenchymal stem cells: comparison of chemokine and growth factor chemotactic activities. Stem Cells 2007;25(7):1737–45.

32. Fiedler J, Röderer G, Günther KP, et al. BMP-2, BMP-4, and PDGF-BB stimulate chemotactic migration of primary human mesenchymal progenitor cells. J Cell Biochem 2002;87(3):305–12.

33. Bouletreau PJ, Warren SM, Spector JA, et al. Factors in the fracture microenvironment induce primary osteoblast angiogenic cytokine production. Plast Reconstr Surg 2002;110(1):139–48.

34. Bergers G, Song S. The role of pericytes in blood-vessel formation and maintenance. Neuro Oncol 2005;7(4):452–64.

35. Smiell JM, Wieman TJ, Steed DL, et al. Efficacy and safety of becaplermin (recombinant human platelet-derived growth factor-BB) in patients with nonhealing, lower extremity diabetic ulcers: a combined analysis of four randomized studies. Wound Repair Regen 1999;7(5):335–46.

36. Margolis DJ, Bartus C, Hoffstad O, et al. Effectiveness of recombinant human platelet-derived growth factor for the treatment of diabetic neuropathic foot ulcers. Wound Repair Regen 2005;13(6):531–6.

37. Nevins M, Giannobile WV, McGuire MK, et al. Platelet-derived growth factor stimulates bone fill and rate of attachment level gain: results of a large multicenter randomized controlled trial. J Periodontol 2005;76(12):2205–15.

38. Lynch SE, Marx RE, Nevins M, et al, editors. Tissue engineering: applications in oral and maxillofacial surgery and periodontics. 2nd edition. Chicago (IL): Quintessence Publishing Company; 2008.

39. Nevins M, Camelo M, Nevins ML, et al. Periodontal regeneration in humans using recombinant human platelet-derived growth factor-BB (rhPDGF-BB) and allogenic bone. J Periodontol 2003;74(9):1282–92.

40. Camelo M, Nevins ML, Schenk RK, et al. Periodontal regeneration in human Class II furcations using purified recombinant human platelet-derived growth factor-BB (rhPDGF-BB) with bone allograft. Int J Periodontics Restorative Dent 2003;23(3): 213–25.

41. Nevins M, Hanratty J, Lynch SE. Clinical results using recombinant human platelet-derived growth factor and mineralized freeze-dried bone allograft in periodontal defects. Int J Periodontics Restorative Dent 2007;27(5):421–7.

42. McGuire MK, Scheyer T, Nevins M, et al. Evaluation of human recession defects treated with coronally advanced flaps and either purified recombinant human platelet-derived growth factor-BB with beta tricalcium phosphate or connective tissue: a histologic and microcomputed tomographic examination. Int J Periodontics Restorative Dent 2009;29(1):7–21.

43. Hollinger JO, Onikepe AO, MacKrell J, et al. Accelerated fracture healing in the geriatric, osteoporotic rat with recombinant human platelet-derived growth factor-BB and an injectable beta-tricalcium phosphate/collagen matrix. J Orthop Res 2008;26(1):83–90.

44. Al-Zube L, Breitbart EA, O'Connor JP, et al. Recombinant human platelet-derived growth factor BB (rhPDGF-BB) and beta-tricalcium phosphate/collagen matrix enhance fracture healing in a diabetic rat model. J Orthop Res 2009;27(8): 1074–81.

45. Moore DC, Ehrlich MG, McAllister SC, et al. Recombinant human platelet-derived growth factor-BB augmentation of new-bone formation in a rat model of distraction osteogenesis. J Bone Joint Surg Am 2009;91(8):1973–84.
46. Coughlin MJ, Grimes JS, Traughber PD, et al. Comparison of radiographs and CT scans in the prospective evaluation of the fusion of hindfoot arthrodesis. Foot Ankle Int 2006;27(10):780–7.
47. Daniels T, DiGiovanni C, Lau JT, et al. Prospective clinical pilot trial in a single cohort of rhPDGF in foot arthrodoses. Foot Ankle Int 2010;31(6):473–9.
48. DiGiovanni CW, Baumhauer J, Lin S, et al. A prospective, randomized, controlled, multi-center human clinical feasibility trial to evaluate the preliminary safety and efficacy of rhPDGF-BB versus autologous bone graft as a bone regeneration device in a foot and ankle fusion model. Foot Ankle Int 2010, in press.
49. DiGiovanni CW, Lin SS, Baumhauer JF, et al. A prospective, randomized, controlled, multi-center pivotal human clinical trial to evaluate the safety and effectiveness of Augment Bone Graft as a substitute for autologous bone. AOFAS Specialty Day Presentation. AAOS Annual Meeting, New Orleans (LA), March 13, 2010.
50. Vaccaro AR, Lawrence JP, Patel T, et al. The safety and efficacy of OP-1 (rhBMP-7) as a replacement for iliac crest autograft in posterolateral lumbar arthrodesis: a long-term (>4 years) pivotal study. Spine (Phila Pa 1976) 2008;33(26):2850–62.
51. Friedlaender GE, Perry CR, Cole JD, et al. Osteogenic protein-1 (bone morphogenetic protein-7) in the treatment of tibial nonunions. J Bone Joint Surg Am 2001; 83(Suppl 1[Pt 2]):S151–8.
52. Cahill KS, Chi JH, Day A, et al. Prevalence, complications, and hospital charges associated with use of bone-morphogenetic proteins in spinal fusion procedures. JAMA 2009;302(1):58–66.
53. Axelrad TW, Einhorn TA. Bone morphogenetic proteins in orthopaedic surgery. Cytokine Growth Factor Rev 2009;20(5–6):481–8.
54. Boakye M, Mummaneni PV, Garrett M, et al. Anterior cervical discectomy and fusion involving a polyetheretherketone spacer and bone morphogenetic protein. J Neurosurg Spine 2005;2(5):521–5.
55. Boraiah S, Paul O, Hawkes D, et al. Complications of recombinant human BMP-2 for treating complex tibial plateau fractures: a preliminary report. Clin Orthop Relat Res 2009;467(12):3257–62.
56. Brower RS, Vickroy NM. A case of psoas ossification from the use of BMP-2 for posterolateral fusion at L4-L5. Spine (Phila Pa 1976) 2008;33(18):E653–5.
57. Deutsch H. High-dose bone morphogenetic protein-induced ectopic abdomen bone growth. Spine J 2010;10(2):e1–4.
58. Joseph V, Rampersaud YR. Heterotopic bone formation with the use of rhBMP2 in posterior minimal access interbody fusion: a CT analysis. Spine (Phila Pa 1976) 2007;32(25):2885–90.
59. Wong DA, Kumar A, Jatana S, et al. Neurologic impairment from ectopic bone in the lumbar canal: a potential complication of off-label PLIF/TLIF use of bone morphogenetic protein-2 (BMP-2). Spine J. 2008;8(6):1011–8.
60. Hee CK, Wisner-Lynch LA, Roden CM, et al. Rotator cuff repair in an ovine model using a combination product comprised of rhPDGF-BB and a type-I bovine collagen matrix. Orthopaedic Research Society Annual Meeting 2010. New Orleans (LA), March, 2010.
61. Hee CK, Roden CM, Wisner-Lynch LA, et al. Evaluation of rhPDGF-BB in combination with a flowable collagen matrix for the treatment of acute Achilles

tendon injury. Orthopaedic Research Society Annual Meeting. New Orleans (LA), March, 2010.

62. Kagel EM, Majeska RJ, Einhorn TA. Effects of diabetes and steroids on fracture healing. Curr Opin Orthop 1995;6(5):7–13.

63. Gerstenfeld LC, Wronski TJ, Hollinger JO, et al. Application of histomorphometric methods to the study of bone repair. J Bone Miner Res 2005;20(10):1715–22.

64. Zhang L, Leeman E, Carnes DC, et al. Human osteoblasts synthesize and respond to platelet-derived growth factor. Am J Physiol 1991;261(2 Pt 1): C348–54.

Platelet-Rich Plasma Concentrate to Augment Bone Fusion

Christopher Bibbo, DO, DPM[a,*], P. Shawn Hatfield, DPM[b]

KEYWORDS

- Foot • Ankle • Bone • Healing • Platelet-rich plasma
- Osteobioligics

Foot and ankle surgeons are often confronted with the challenge of obtaining satisfactory bone healing, in a timely fashion, in patients with multiple risk factors for poor bony healing. Despite the recent sports press media attention to platelet-rich plasma (PRP), the practicing musculoskeletal surgeon and particularly the foot and ankle surgeon have long used PRP to assist with bone healing. The widespread application of PRP stems from the work of Marx and colleagues[1] in the field of oral-maxillofacial surgery. The sentinel original work of these investigators, and that of Urist, heralded the onset of the era of orthobiologic augmentation to enhance bone healing. The application of PRP to augment bone healing subsequently spread to the field of spine and orthopedic surgery, generating both basic science efforts and clinical evaluations of platelet (PLT)-derived growth factors on bone healing. Despite a large body of basic science and clinical work in the oral maxillofacial literature that firmly supports the clinical utility of PRP, the body of research and basic science within the spine literature appears to be split on the utility of PRP. However, an area of musculoskeletal surgery that deals with a high frequency of patient encounters at risk for bone healing problems and possessing multiple cumulative risk factors for bone healing is foot and ankle surgery (**Box 1**). Ironically, within the foot and ankle literature, there exists only a handful of basic science and clinical articles reporting on the efficacy and clinical utility of PRP. This article of *Foot and Ankle Clinics of North America* discusses the concept and basic science of PRP, and clinical applications of PRP for the augmentation of bone healing in foot and ankle surgery. The authors also provide a classification system that assesses relative risks for poor bone healing and the need for orthobiologic augmentation.

[a] Foot and Ankle Section, Department of Orthopaedics, Marshfield Clinic, 1000 North Oak Avenue, Marshfield, WI 54449, USA
[b] Podiatry Associates of Indiana, 5471 Georgetown Road Suite C, Indianapolis, IN 46234, USA
* Corresponding author.
E-mail address: cbibbo@charter.net

Foot Ankle Clin N Am 15 (2010) 641–649
doi:10.1016/j.fcl.2010.09.002
1083-7515/10/$ – see front matter © 2010 Elsevier Inc. All rights reserved.

Box 1
Summary of risk factors for poor bone healing (partial list)

- Smoking
- Diabetes and Charcot
- History of high-energy injury
- Multiple surgeries at osseous surgical site
- History of delayed/nonunion
- History of avascular necrosis
- Alcohol abuse
- Immunosuppression
- Acute, uncontrolled infections
- Chronic infections
- Poor soft tissue envelope
- Suboptimal vascularity
- Collagen disorders
- Multiple medical comorbidities
- Irradiation to surgical site

Plus more...

BASIC SCIENCE OF PRP

PRP, derived from autologous blood, is defined as a volume of plasma with a PLT concentration typically 5 times greater than physiologic levels (≈ 1 million/mL). PLTs typically possess any number of growth factors within the confines of the cell membrane, namely in the alpha-granules. Upon degranulation, PLTs release these growth factors, many of which are involved in healing cascades (**Box 2**).[2] Increases in levels of growth factors have been clearly demonstrated to correlate with

---

Box 2
Key growth factors contained in PRP: basic function in bone healing

- Platelet derived growth factor (PDGF): chemotaxis, mitogenesis, differentiation of osteoprogenitor cells, (+) autocrine feedback on cytokines/growth factors
- Transforming growth factor-β (TGF-β): chemotaxis, mitogenesis, mesenchymal cell differentiation (chondrocyte phenotype)
- Epidermal growth factor (EGF): *mitogenesis*
- Insulinlike growth factor (IGF): chemotaxis, cell proliferation, cell differentiation of mesenchymal stem cells/periosteal cells/osteoblasts/chondrocytes
- Vascular endothelial growth factor (VEGF): *chemotaxis*
- Seratonin (5HT): potential osteoblast mitogen
- Thrombospondin-1: potential regulator of angiogenesis in bone healing
- Basic fibroblast growth factor (FGF2): potential positive influence on marrow stromal cells (preosteoblasts)

---

increasingly higher PLT concentrations with postrelease concentrations ranging from 300% to 500% higher than normal homeostatic levels.[3] Clinically, nonunions have been demonstrated to be devoid of these growth factors.[4] It is now generally accepted that PRP acts as a reservoir of several critical growth factors involved in the healing cascade, including that of bone repair (see **Box 2**). A recent study found some additional interesting data: when compared with human bone reamings harvested in vivo for grafting procedures, PRP demonstrated higher levels of vascular endothelial growth factor (VEGF), PLT-derived growth factor (PDGF), insulinlike growth factor (IGF)-I, and transforming growth factor (TGF)-beta1.[5] These data further support the theory of PRP as a reservoir for critical bone-healing growth factors.

In vitro, PRP has been demonstrated to exert a dose-dependent increase in mitogenesis and chemotaxis on mesenchymal stem cells[6] and a profound effect on committed osteogenic cells, promoting a 50-fold mitogenic response on fetal osteoblasts, that may last for nearly 2 months.[7] In contrast, a recent paper determined that in vitro, PRP may impair the development of osteoclasts, with this effect becoming more profound with exposure to increasing levels of PRP to incubated osteoclast precursor cells.[8] In vivo, in the athymic and diabetic rat models, PRP has shown to improve bone interface characteristics.[9] An important finding by Weibrech and colleagues[10] is that PRP may have either an inhibitor effect at low (270,000/μL) and very high (2.5 million/μL) PLT levels, but exert a positive effect at a PLT concentration of approximately 1 million/μL. Herein lies a potential confounding factor at the point of care: if PLT levels are not maintained (ostensibly diminished by "wash-out" or edema), PRP may actually result in a deleterious effect. It is the authors' opinion that the aforementioned provides a potential partial explanation for mixed results in the spine literature on PRP.

Evidenced-Based Medicine on PRP to Augment Bone Healing in Foot and Ankle Surgery

The first reported use of PRP in foot and ankle surgery was performed by S.S. Lin and colleagues at New Jersey Medical School in the treatment of closed ankle fractures. In this prospective study, all patients had undergone a single operation for treatment of the ankle fracture and ranged in age from 18 to 72 years. All patients received surgery within 20 days of the ankle injury. The purpose of the study was to evaluate the treatment of ankle fracture nonunion site with PRP and standard internal fixation techniques. Duration of nonunion ranged from 2 to 6 months and the mean patient age was 42 years. The findings of this prospective study showed successful union achieved at a mean time of 8.5 weeks.[4] These investigators also compared plasma and fracture hematoma growth factor concentrations in patients with nonunions versus those with acute fractures. In examining the level of growth factors found in the plasma, a significant reduction of plasma PDGF and plasma TGF-beta were noted in nonunion patients. Even more notable was a significant reduction in fracture hematoma PDGF and TGF-beta in patients with nonunions compared with the fresh fracture population. The conclusion of their study clearly indicates that the fractures that progressed to nonunion exhibited a significant reduction in both plasma and fracture site PDGF and TGF-beta. The addition of PRP, with the release of platelet granules, provides important growth factors and initiation of cytokine autocrine feedback loops, resulting in a positive impact on bone healing.

To date, the only Level I evidence study on PRP in foot and ankle surgery has been from the Marshfield Clinic by Bibbo and colleagues.[11] In this single-surgeon study, the investigators analyzed the clinical and radiologic results, as well as complications, after the use of adjuvant PRP in high-risk patients undergoing elective foot and ankle surgery. Sixty-two high-risk patients were prospectively enrolled, totaling 123 operative procedures, mostly fusions. The mean patient age was 51 years (range 16–76; the gender distribution was slightly more females). All patients possessed risk factors for bone healing, including diabetes and smoking (37%); nearly 70% of patients possessed multiple risk factors for poor bone healing.

This study used bone graft only when required to fill a bone void or defect. Patients were prospectively evaluated for time to union and complications. The investigators reported a mean overall time to union of 41 days. The data were further scrutinized to evaluate union time and fusion rate according to anatomic location. The investigators reported a significant difference when comparing hindfoot/ankle fusions versus forefoot fusions. Ankle procedures had mean time to union of 40 days with an overall union rate of 95%. This was comparable to patients receiving hindfoot procedures, which were noted to have a mean time to fusion of 43 days and union rate of 92%. Similar findings were seen with midfoot procedures. Forefoot procedures exhibited mean time to fusion of 38 days with 100% union rate. The study also noted no significant improvement in time to fusion when PRP was combined with autograft (45 days with PRP plus autograft vs 40 days with PRP alone). A brief comparison of these results to implantable DC stimulators showed an improved time to union and increased union rate with lower reported complication rate than that noted in the literature with implantable DC stimulators.

The second variable evaluated in the use of PRP in high-risk foot and ankle patients was complications associated with the use of PRP. The most common complication encountered was infection. Infection tended to occur in patients with diabetes, Charcot arthropathy, skin ulcerations, and collagen vascular disease. Some of the deep infections occurred in a stable osseous setting with fusion noted on radiographs. These deep infections were a result of delayed wound healing and contiguous spread of the inoculum. No complications were associated with the handling or harvesting of PRP. The investigators concluded adjunctive use of PRP in high-risk elective foot and ankle surgery results in acceptable time to union with low reported rates of complications. The use of PRP does not negate the importance of surgical technique, and proper joint surface preparation and fixation in obtaining good surgical outcomes.

A third study on PRP by Coetzee[12] examined the application of PRP in foot and ankle surgery as an ancillary data collection on the Agility total ankle replacement (TAR).[13] The study compared the syndesmotic fusion rates using PRP-augmented bone grafting versus a control of non–PRP-augmented bone grafting during TAR surgery. This retrospective evaluation compared 66 patients augmented with PRP with 114 historical controls. Serial radiographs were performed. If no clear radiographic evidence of fusion was noted, a CT scan was obtained to evaluate for nonunion. A fusion rate of 61% was noted in the control arm of the study at 8 weeks postoperatively and 85% after 6 months. The remaining 15% of the patients were then classified as delayed or nonunion depending on radiographic appearance. In contrast, syndesmotic fusion rates during TAR using PRP-augmented bone graft resulted in a 76% union rate at 8 weeks, 18% more achieved union at 3 months, and an additional 3% union rate at 6 months for an overall fusion rate of 97%. This study shows a statistical significance in the use of PRP-augmented bone grafting during syndesmotic fusion when compared with non–PRP-augmented bone grafting. An important analysis comparing nonunion rates of smoking patients was also performed. Of those patients in the control arm, a 50% fusion rate at 6 months was noted compared with an 80% fusion rate at 6 months in the PRP-augmented patient population. Improved overall time to fusion was also noted in the PRP-augmented fusions. This study illustrates the improvement of fusion rates in smoking patients and overall reduction in time to fusion in patients receiving PRP-augmented bone grafting.

When comparing the dental, spine, and foot and ankle literature on the use of PRP to augment bone healing, it is evident that there exists a disparity in results. The limited number of foot and ankle articles has positive results, similar to that of the dental literature, whereas the spine literature has split results. It is quite possible that this discrepancy is related to the physiologic and mechanical differences experienced by the local anatomy, differences in implant/instrumentation, the particular surgical needs, and quite possibly, pushing PRP beyond its role as an adjuvant.

PRP BONE TECHNIQUES

One of the advantages of PRP is that it is designed for the point of care in the operating room. In general, 2 techniques may be used with PRP: traditional open, and percutaneous technique of Lin. Both open and percutaneous techniques require the preparation of PRP. Although no universally accepted "standardized" technique for the preparation of PRP exists, a few particulars are noteworthy. Typically, PRP is prepared by harvest of the patient's own peripheral blood as close in time as possible to the moment where PRP is desired. No studies have clearly demonstrated the superiority of arterial versus venous blood draws for PRP production; the attendant risks of arterial blood draws are more obvious. Venous blood harvest requires attention to proper needle size to prevent fluid shear and subsequent cell crenation and early degranulation. Next, blood is immediately treated with an anticoagulant. Sodium citrate appears to be "gentler" to PLTs than EDTA, but both appear to provide adequate anticlotting function in the preparation of PRP. Next, the blood sample is centrifuged, generally at a force of $200g$ for 10 minutes, separating red cells from PLTs. A second centrifuge process then extracts the remaining aqueous phase, yielding a PLT "pellet" as the centrifugate. The PLT pellet is then resuspended into a "gel" medium that is delivered to the operative site. Thrombin, within a particular range, along with calcium chloride, is required for the optimum degranulation (activation) of platelets (142.8 U/mL bovine thrombin, 14.3 mg/mL $CaCl_2$).[13] The use of bovine thrombin to create the PLT gel has been implicated with antibody production with the risk of inducing a coagulopathy; newer gelling agents may avert this risk.[14] Each manufacturer has particular methodology for the preparation of PRP, but all follow the same basic protocol. No study has clearly proven superiority of one manufacturer's PRP production device over another; however, industry claims exist of improved PLT yield and improved PLT condition with each proprietor's device. Clinically, the lead author Christopher Bibbo has observed failure of certain proprietary PRP systems because of premature admixture of PLTs and thrombin/$CaCl_2$, resulting in premature PLT activation, sludging within the PRP delivery system, and suboptimal system performance. Generally, steps can be taken intraoperatively to mitigate these problems, and manufacturers have been responsive to these issues.

In the traditional open technique, after PRP is prepared, the PRP product is dispensed (typically sprayed) onto opposing native bony surfaces or bone graft surfaces (typically allograft). After a gel-like coagulum is in place, it is not mobilized or washed away with irrigation fluid—final irrigation of the operative field must be performed before the application of PRP. The surgical incisions are then closed in the usual fashion. The use of drains has been debated among clinicians, theorizing the removal of PRP in a closed suction drain system. This is, however, unlikely and unproven, and drains should be used as needed. Platelet-poor plasma (the supernatant derived in the PRP centrifugation process) is rich in pro-coagulants and is often used to promote hemostasis at wound closure.

Dr Sheldon Lin has clinically used an alternative technique to the open surgical application of PRP. Dr Lin's technique is a percutaneous technique in which PRP can be applied to impending nonunions and delayed unions, especially in at-risk patients through a minimally invasive approach (unpublished data). Under fluoroscopy, the suspect bone site is identified; a miniature incision is placed, through which debridement may be accomplished; PRP is then introduced percutaneously directly into the bony site, followed by skin closure. This delivery technique, although not yet published as a "surgical technique" or quantified in a robust prospective study, finds significant daily clinical utility in difficult clinical situations where limited incisions and minimally invasive techniques are desired, such as in diabetic ankle fractures.

Who Is an Appropriate Candidate for PRP: Which Patient, When, and Why?

When assessing each individual patient for the need of orthobiologic augmentation, the authors categorize each patient for the risk of poor bone healing based on specific medical risks (comorbidities), as well as the condition of the bone at the proposed surgical site (**Fig. 1**). The particular surgical goal (eg, bone defect spanning vs simple osteotomy), as well as the specific surgical indication for that patient's particular operation, is also weighed. As it is clear that emerging data are demonstrating that each orthobiologic agent is not equal, the authors have created a "host" surgical site classification system to assess the need of orthobiologic augmentation. This classification system is based on specific physiologic characteristics of each patient and creates risk factors for delayed and nonunions as well as the actual physical characteristics of the surgical site in question. These variables impart a separate and distinct but comorbid set of characteristics that are determined by the quality of the bone at the surgical site as well as the soft tissue envelope and the particular requirement of the surgical intervention. As described in the authors' classification system, the need

"1-A" Host-Surgical Site Good Host Good Surgical Site Bone*	"1-B" Host-Surgical Site Good Host Bad Surgical Site Bone*
"2-A" Host-Surgical Site Bad Host* Good Surgical Site Bone	"2-B" Host-Surgical Site Bad host* Bad Surgical Site Bone*

(* = add-up the number of contributing medical co-morbidities & surgical site risk

factors to obtain a relative-weighted risk scale)

Fig. 1. Bibbo host-surgical site classification system to assess bone-healing risk.

for orthobiologic augmentation increases with the severity of the problem. Thus, as can be gleamed from this surgical classification (see **Fig. 1; Fig. 2**), the need for orthobiologic augmentation in a relatively young healthy patient with a clean, elective minor surgical procedure is low. However, on the other end of the spectrum, a patient possessing multiple premorbid physiologic characteristics of poor bone healing, along with a proposed surgical site that creates a local environment not suitable for bone healing, imparts a completely different set of characteristics in which orthobiologic augmentation is likely to be sought by the surgeon in addition to any allograft or autograft. As can be seen, the host surgical site classification system (Bibbo) also portends along its spectrum the potential use of different orthobiologic augmentations (see **Fig. 1**). For example, in patients who have limited risk factors and surgical sites that convey a lower level of properties that would contribute to bony healing problems, PRP may be an appropriate adjunct to fusions (see **Fig. 1**). In comparison, a patient with multiple medical comorbidities and a relatively dysvascular surgical site with a poor soft tissue envelope would impart the need for a more robust orthobiologic augmentation agent, such as bone morphogenetic protein-2.

Practical Clinical Considerations

One of the benefits of PRP is that it is readily available: PRP preparations can be considered a transfusion technique performed and delivered at the point of care. Thus, no special requirement above that of patient consent and the ability to draw blood and the availability of a particular proprietary PLT concentrating system are required for its use. For the outpatient setting, where the most common surgical procedures are performed, PRP is readily available. It should be noted the application of PRP is no longer a billable service in the United States. However, this should not dissuade the surgeon from using PRP when he or she feels it is clinically in the patient's best interest. On the other hand, the ready availability of PRP to the general practicing musculoskeletal surgeon has rendered a tide of activity that has attempted to use PRP to cover all the bases as a biologic augmentation when indeed it may not be the most appropriate agent. For example, in the lead author's Christopher Bibbo's referral practice, there has been the observation of the use of PRP as a lone, freestanding agent in an to attempt to heal bony surgical sites in patients with multiple complex comorbidities. It is the authors' opinion that the use of PRP as the singular orthobiologic agent is not appropriate. These patients may require extensive grafting and orthobiologic augmentation with more robust agents. Once again, it is the authors' opinion that when failure of PRP is observed in these complex patients, a generalized perception of inefficacy is made regarding the value of PRP. A vested understanding of when PRP should be used is very important. PRP has the potential to help augment bony healing in what we would consider the less complex surgical

Host-Surgical Site Class	Adjuvant Need
"1-A" Host-Surgical Site *(favorable for bone healing)* -------------	[+ / -]
"1-B" Host-Surgical Site *(not favorable)* -----------------------------	[+]
"2-A" Host-Surgical Site *(bad)* ---	[+ +]
"2-B" Host-Surgical Site *(worse)* ---------------------------------------	[+ + +]

Fig. 2. Relative osteobiologic adjuvant need based on the Bibbo host-surgical site classification system.

reconstructions. When considering the use of PRP, there are no data to suggest that the addition of other "pro-osteogenic" graft materials (other than bone) will act synergistically with PRP. In fact, one study suggests that certain bone graft substitute materials (eg, tricalcium phosphate) may actually result in poorer results when mixed with PRP versus PRP alone.[15]

SUMMARY

The community-based foot and ankle surgeon often treats patients with significant comorbidities and local tissue pathology, which makes osseous procedures, and in particular arthrodeses, substantially more difficult. A complete understanding of orthobiologic augmentation products available to the surgeon is crucial in assisting the surgeon to successfully apply these technologies and help to ensure improved surgical outcomes. PRP offers a relatively cost-efficient method of delivering directly to the surgical site a number of key growth factors known to be instrumental in the bone-healing cascade. In the United States, many community-based practitioners often find their "hands tied" when it comes to the use of expensive biologic materials in both the hospital and surgical center settings. The body of evidence on the use of PRP in the foot and ankle literature is small, but compelling, with a greater amount of positive data existing in the dental and spine literature. It appears that relative proportions of PLTs in PRP may be critical to the successful application of PRP. Despite the limited number of foot and ankle PRP studies, it is the authors' opinion that PRP provides a safe and cost-effective method of delivering important growth factors to promote osseous healing in patients at moderate risk for delayed and nonunion. Nothing eliminates the need for appropriate surgical indications and meticulous surgical technique; PRP is, strictly speaking, an orthobiologic *adjuvant* that may be used to assist with bone healing.

REFERENCES

1. Marx RE, Carlson ER, Eichstaedt RM, et al. Platelet-rich plasma growth factor enhancement for bone grafts. Oral Surg Oral Med Oral Pathol Oral Radiol Endod 1998;85:638–46.
2. Kevy S, Jacobsen M, Kadiyala S. Characterization of growth factor levels in platelet concentrates. 5th Annual Hilton Head Workshop on Engineering Tissues. February 2002.
3. Babbush CA, Kevy SV, Jacobson MS. An in vitro and in vivo evaluation of autologous platelet concentrate in oral reconstruction. Implant Dent 2003;12:24–34.
4. Gandhi A, Van Gelderen J, Berberian WS, et al. Platelet releasate enhances healing in patients with a non-union. Chicago: Orthopaedic Research Society; 2003.
5. Schmidmaier G, Herrmann S, Green J, et al. Quantitative assessment of growth factors in reaming aspirate, iliac crest, and platelet preparation. Bone 2006; 39(5):1156–63.
6. Haynseworth S, Kadiyala L, Liang L, et-al. Chemotactic and mitogenic stimulation of human mesenchymal stem cells by platelet rich plasma suggests a mechanism for bone repair. 48th Annual Meeting of the orthopaedic Research Society. Dallas (TX), 2002.
7. Slater M, Patava K, Klingham K, et al. Involvement of platelets in stimulating osteogenic activity. J Orthop Res 1995;13:655–63.
8. Cenni E, Avnet S, Fotia C, et al. Platelet-rich plasma impairs osteoclast generation from human precursors of peripheral blood. J Orthop Res 2010;28(6):792–7.

9. Siebrecht MA, De Rooij PP, Arm DM, et al. Platelet concentrate increases bone ingrowth into porous hydroxyapatite. Orthopedics 2001;25:169–72.
10. Weibrech G, Hansen T, Kleis W, et al. Effect of platelet concentration in platelet-rich plasma on peri-implant bone regeneration. Bone 2004;34:665–71.
11. Bibbo C, Bono CM, Lin SS. Union rates using autologous platelet concentrate alone and with bone graft in high-risk foot & ankle surgery patients. J Surg Orthop Adv 2005;14:17–22.
12. Coetzee C. The use of autologous concentrated growth factors to promote syndesmosis fusion in the agility total ankle replacement. A preliminary study. Foot Ankle Int 2005;26:840–6.
13. Gandi A, Bibbo C, Pinzur M, et al. The role of platelet-rich plasma in foot & ankle surgery. Foot Ankle Clin 2005;10:621–37.
14. Lacoste E, Martineau J, Gagnon G. Platelet concentrates: effects of calcium and thrombin on endothelial cell proliferation and growth factor release. J Periodontol 2003;74:1498–507.
15. Butcher A, Milner R, Ellis K, et al. Interaction of platelet-rich concentrate with bone graft materials: an in vitro study. J Orthop Trauma 2009;23:195–200.

Shock Wave Therapy as a Treatment of Nonunions, Avascular Necrosis, and Delayed Healing of Stress Fractures

John P. Furia, MD[a],*, Jan D. Rompe, MD[b], Angelo Cacchio, MD[c],
Nicola Maffulli, MD, MS, PhD, FRCS(Orth), FFSEM(UK)[d]

KEYWORDS

• Shock wave therapy • Nonunion • Avascular necrosis
• Stress fracture

Shock wave therapy (SWT) is most commonly used to treat soft tissue conditions such as tendinopathies and fasciopathies. However, SWT was originally described as a treatment of pathologic conditions of bone. In 1988, German investigators observed an increase in pelvic bone formation in patients treated with shock waves during lithotripsy procedures.[1] Soon after, Valchanou and Michailov[2] reported on successful use of high-energy shock waves in the treatment of delayed fractures and nonunions. Subsequent clinical trials performed at European and Asian centers have also yielded favorable results.[3–8]

In the United States, SWT is rarely used to treat disorders of bone. Many of the landmark basic science and clinical trials have been performed in centers outside the United States.[3–30] Some of this work has been published in non-English journals.[29,30] Perhaps for these reasons, many physicians in the United States are unfamiliar with how SWT can be used to treat pathologic conditions of bone such as nonunions, avascular necrosis (AVN), and delayed healing of stress fractures.

[a] SUN Orthopedics and Sports Medicine, Department of Orthopedic Surgery, 900 Buffalo Road, Lewisburg, PA 17837, USA
[b] OrthoTrauma Evaluation Center, Department of Orthopedics, Oppenheimer Street 70, D-55130 Mainz, Germany
[c] Department of Physical Medicine and Rehabilitation, University of Rome "La Sapienza", Rome, Italy
[d] Centre for Sports and Exercise Medicine, Department of Orthopedics, Barts and the London School of Medicine and Dentistry, London, Great Britain, UK
* Corresponding author.
E-mail address: jfuria@ptd.net

Foot Ankle Clin N Am 15 (2010) 651–662
doi:10.1016/j.fcl.2010.07.002
1083-7515/10/$ – see front matter © 2010 Elsevier Inc. All rights reserved.

At present, the Food and Drug Administration has approved shock wave generators for use in soft tissue indications (plantar fasciopathy and lateral epicondylitis) only.[31,32] The scarcity of shock wave generating devices, availability of other treatment options, variations in treatment protocols, and reimbursement issues have also had a negative effect on the adaptation of this procedure. Collectively, these obstacles explain why SWT is rarely used in the United States to treat disorders of bone.

Yet SWT has many advantages over other forms of treatment, including its comparative safety, low complication rate, and ease of patient compliance. Although there are some conflicting reports, there are now many published clinical trials that support the use of SWT as a treatment of nonunion, AVN, and stress fractures.[3–6,26,33–40]

The aim of this review is to describe some of the ways SWT can be used to treat common disorders of bone. After a consideration of some basic concepts, this review focuses on how SWT is currently used to treat nonunions, AVN, and stress fractures.

SWT BASIC PRINCIPLES

In physics, a shock wave is defined as an acoustic sound wave characterized by a high peak pressure (up to 500 bar), a fast initial increase time of less than 10 ns, a short life cycle (<10 ms), and a broad frequency spectrum (16–20 MHz).[31,41,42]

Shock waves are produced by commercially available shock wave generators. Shock wave production is device specific. Depending on the device, electromagnetically, electrohydraulically, piezoelectrically, or electropneumatically derived energy is transformed into a shock wave.[31,41,42] Each device concentrates the shock waves so that they can be applied in sufficient quantity to stimulate a desired tissue response.[31,42]

Such focused shock waves are transmitted to a small area (the focus), and the maximum energy is delivered several centimeters below the skin.[31,42]

Radial shock waves are produced by more recently developed pneumatic devices. Radial shock waves transfer their maximum energy more superficially, at or just below the skin surface, and distribute the energy radially into the treated tissues.[43]

The physical properties of a shock wave are similar regardless of the method of production. For clinical use, the shock waves are applied directly to tissues using the shock wave generator's targeting device. The waves are dispersed from the application site and then may be absorbed, reflected, or dissipated depending on the properties of the particular tissue.[31,42]

Shock waves have both a direct and indirect effect on treated tissues.[31,40] The absorbed shock waves produce a tensile force, and this tensile force accounts for the direct effect.[31] Shock waves also stimulate the formation of cavitation bubbles.[31,42] The bubbles expand, contract, collide, and form other bubbles in the treated tissues.[31,44] The resulting energy also stimulates a biologic response, the so-called indirect effect.[31,42]

PARAMETERS

The biologic effects of SWT on the musculoskeletal system are parameter specific.[27,28,44] SWT is generally safe. However, excessive shock wave energy can result in irreversible cellular damage.[27,28,44] Not all protocols are effective, and a protocol that is effective for one indication may not be effective for another. For these reasons, a working knowledge of the critical treatment parameters is paramount to achieving a good result.

Before considering specific treatment parameters, it is first necessary to distinguish between high-energy (>0.2 mJ/mm^2) and low-energy (<0.2 mJ/mm^2) SWT. High-energy SWT usually consists of 1 or 2 treatments performed in an operating room or ambulatory surgical center with some form of anesthesia. High-energy treatments are usually used when treating deeper structures, tend to be more painful than low-energy treatments, and are commonly used to treat disorders of bone. Low-energy SWT is typically performed in multiple sessions.[2–4] Low-energy treatments are usually, but not always, used for more superficial structures, need no form of anesthesia, and are commonly used when treating tendinopathy, fasciopathy, and more superficially located bones. At present, there are no published randomized controlled clinical trials comparing outcomes of high- and low-energy SWT for the treatment of disorders of bone.

The critical treatment parameters include the total amount of energy per treatment, number of shocks per session, frequency of shocks, energy per shock, number of treatments, and interval between treatments. Each parameter can be manipulated to modulate the clinical response.

The term energy flux density (EFD) refers to the amount of energy in a given amount of tissue (usually mm^2) at a given point in time.[34,40] EFD is a standard method of quantifying the total amount of energy delivered in a treatment session. EFD is simply the product of the energy per shock and the number of shocks and is expressed in the unit millijoule per area.

High- and low-energy sessions can yield equivalent EFD. For example, a high-energy session using an energy level of 0.3 mJ/mm^2 and 1000 shocks and a low-energy session using 0.1 mJ/mm^2 and 3000 shocks yield an equivalent EFD of 300 mJ/mm^2 each.

The number of shocks, interval between shocks, number of treatments, and interval between treatments are additional parameters that can determine the therapeutic response.[28,31,44] Like energy, the parameters are easily manipulated, and this manipulation, in part, explains why protocols used to treat the same condition can vary significantly.

BIOLOGIC RESPONSE TO SWT

Recent histologic, biochemical, and immunologic basic science studies have greatly advanced the understanding of how shock waves affect treated tissues.[9–11,13,14,18–25,44,45] These effects include enhanced neovascularity, accelerated growth factor release, selective neural inhibition, osteogenic stem cell recruitment, and inhibition of molecules that have a role in inflammation.[9–11,13,14,18–25,44,45] Enhanced neovascularity, increased growth factor release, and accentuated osteogenic stem cell recruitment are probably the most important effects on bone and are therefore the focus of this section.

SWT upregulates the expression of proteins and growth factors that are critical for angiogenesis. Wang and colleagues[20] reported on the effect of low-energy SWT on neovascularization at the tendon-bone junction in rabbits. Bone-tendon junctions treated with low-energy SWT had higher number of neovessels and angiogenesis-related markers, including endothelial nitric oxide synthase, vascular endothelial growth factor (VEGF), and proliferating cell nuclear antigen, than the untreated controls.[20] Of note, VEGF is an important mitogenic factor for vascular endothelial cells,[36] and endothelial cell proliferation is a critical aspect of angiogenesis.

Ma and colleagues,[22] using a rabbit model, examined the effects of SWT on femoral heads with AVN. They also noted enhanced VEGF and messenger RNA (mRNA)-VEGF expression in the treated specimens.

In a subsequent animal trial by the same investigators, SWT was shown to upregulate the growth factor bone morphogenic protein 2 (BMP-2) and its mRNA. BMP-2 is an important mediator of bone formation and bone remodeling.[23]

In regard to osteogenesis, Wang and colleagues[19] noted increased BMD, increased callus formation, increased ash content, and increase calcium content in specimens treated with high-energy SWT. Subsequent mechanical studies showed that the treated bone had enhanced strength, significantly higher peak load to failure, higher peak stress, and greater elasticity when compared with controls.[19]

The same investigators also noted selective destruction of osteocytes and microfractures of bony trabeculae in rabbits treated with SWT.[13] Approximately 3 weeks after treatment, histologic and biochemical analysis revealed thickening of the cortex, increase in the number of bony trabeculae, and a significant increase in the number and activity of treated osteoblasts.[13]

In still another study, Maier and colleagues[45] used a rabbit model to demonstrate that application of shock waves with an EFD of 0.5 mJ/mm^2 resulted in new periosteal bone formation in treated femurs.

To summarize, SWT seems to produce its effects on bone by upregulating proteins critical for angiogenesis, accentuating the release of growth factors important in osteogenesis, and stimulating the production of osteoblasts. Additional studies are necessary to sort out the relative importance of each of these effects.

PROCEDURE
Management of Disorders of Bone

The procedure for SWT in disorders of bone is similar to that used in soft tissues disorders. Deeper structures are treated with high energy, whereas more superficial pathologic conditions may be treated with either a high- or low-energy protocol.

The pathologic area is carefully examined, and the area of maximal pain and tenderness is identified. This so-called clinical focusing, as opposed to simply relying on image guidance, has been shown in clinical trials to improve outcomes of SWT.[46,47] Clinical focusing is often, but not always, supplemented with image guidance to assure that the shock waves are applied to the area of intended treatment.

Ultrasound gel is applied to the skin overlying the bone. The targeting arm of the shock wave generator is then placed in contact with the gel-prepared skin. The targeting device is aimed in such a way that the administered shock waves are directed at the fracture site.

The shock waves are applied in a dynamic manner. Treatment usually begins centrally, at the point of maximal tenderness, and then proceeds circumferentially, so that all the pathologic tissues are treated. The average size of the treatment area varies with the size of the bone and is usually several centimeters in length and width.

Specific Disorders of Bones

Nonunions
Even with the recent advances in fracture care, fracture nonunion remains a challenging clinical problem. Treatment is often highly individualized, complex, and demanding.

Nonoperative management using some type of immobilization, restricted weight bearing, pharmacologic intervention, pulsed electrotherapy, or a combination of all can be successful. However, compliance with these forms of treatment is often difficult. Other potential problems include continued pain in spite of radiographic osteosynthesis, significant muscle atrophy, disuse osteoporosis, increased susceptibility to reinjury, and perhaps most significantly, persistent fracture nonunion.[48–53]

Although attractive, more novel procedures such as bone growth stimulation with pulsed electric therapy, low-intensity ultrasonography, and orthobiologic enhancement with recombinant osteogenic protein and growth factors have yielded inconsistent results.[54–58] For this reason, most clinicians recommend a surgical approach.[50–52] Usually, surgical approach involves some type of autogenous or allogenic bone grafting procedure with some form of internal or external fixation. These procedures can be lengthy and difficult; significant morbidity and complications are not uncommon.[49,51,53]

Warren and Brooker[59] reported an infection rate of 13% in patients undergoing surgical treatment of chronic nonunion. Younger and Chapman[60] reported a 9% incidence of serious complications including deep infection, persistent drainage, hematoma, neurovascular injury, and pain persisting for more than 6 months postoperation.

Acknowledging the prolonged healing time and prevalence of persistent nonunion associated with some forms of traditional nonoperative management as well as the potential complications and morbidity associated with surgical intervention, additional treatment methods are desirable. SWT has shown some promise. In a systematic review of the use of SWT as a treatment of nonunion, Birnbaum and colleagues[33] identified 10 high-quality studies involving a total of 631 patients and reported a healing rate of 75% to 91%.[33]

Procedure The procedure is typically performed on an outpatient basis with a high-energy protocol using monitored anesthesia care, sedation, or a regional block.

Patients are positioned in a supine position on a radiolucent fracture table. The fracture site is localized with an image intensifier or ultrasonographic device. Ultrasound gel is applied to the skin overlying the site of the nonunion. The center of the shock wave targeting device (the focal point) was positioned in such a way that the administered shock waves are directed at the fracture site. The targeting device is then docked to the skin overlying the nonunion site. Shock waves are applied to the fracture nonunion site and the adjacent cortical structures from an anteroposterior direction. The average size of the treatment area varies with the size of the bone, but is usually several centimeters in width and length. The procedure is guided using the image intensifier.

Nonunions are usually treated with 2000 to 6000 shocks using an EFD between 0.3 mJ/mm^2 and 0.6 mJ/mm^2. The total number of impulses is usually divided along the proximal and distal margins of the nonunion. Treatments typically last approximately 10 to 20 minutes. The total number of treatments (typically ranging from 1–4) and the interval between treatments (typically ranging from 1–4 weeks) vary from center to center.

After completion of the procedure, the extremity is assessed for swelling hematoma and ecchymosis, which are rare. Fracture pattern, location, stability, and discretion of the physician often determine if and how a treated limb will be immobilized. Patients are usually monitored the same day in the surgery recovery area and then discharged later that day.

Results Animal nonunion models have been used to study the effects of high-energy SWT on cortical bone.[12] In a canine nonunion trial, all of the treated subjects reached radiographically observable bony union 12 weeks after the shock wave treatment, whereas untreated control subjects had radiographically persistent nonunions at termination of the study.[12]

Several large European and Asian trauma centers routinely use SWT to treat nonunions.[3-6] Results of uncontrolled clinical trials have been promising.[3,4,6] Schaden and colleagues[3] reported on 115 patients with nonunions or delayed unions of various fractures who were treated with high-energy SWT and immobilization. Follow-up ranged from 3 months to 4 years.[3] Overall, 87 patients (75.7%) were reported to have healed fractures.[3]

Rompe and colleagues[6] reported their experience using high-energy SWT to treat 43 patients with either a tibial or femoral diaphyseal nonunion. They noted bony consolidation in 31 of 43 cases (72%) after an average of 4 months posttreatment.[6]

Wang and colleagues[4] used high-energy SWT as a treatment of 72 nonunions of long-bone fractures. A 12-month follow-up was available for 55 patients.[4] For the entire cohort, an overall healing rate of 80% (44 of 55 patients) was noted.[4]

Cachio and colleagues,[5] in a randomized clinical trial, compared 3 groups of patients. Groups 1 and 2 received SWT (4 treatments of 4000 shocks) with an EFD of 0.4 mJ/mm^2 and 0.7 mJ/mm^2, respectively.[5] Patients in group 3 were treated with surgery.[5] The patients in the 3 groups had similar demographic characteristics.[5] At 6 months postintervention, 70% of nonunions in group 1, 71% of nonunions in group 2, and 73% of nonunions in group 3 had healed.[5] It was concluded that SWT was as effective as surgery in stimulating union of long-bone nonunions.[5]

The efficacy of SWT as a treatment of nonunions depends on the type of nonunion (atrophic or hypertrophic).[4,7] Haupt[7] reported a 100% healing rate among 27 patients with hypertrophic nonunions compared with only 23% (3 of 13 patients) with atrophic nonunions. Wang and colleagues[4] reported a success rate of 80% for patients with hypertrophic nonunions versus only 27% for patients with atrophic nonunions.

Xu and colleagues[8] reported an overall healing rate of 75.4% in their series of 69 nonunions (22 femurs, 28 tibias, 13 humeri, 5 radiuses, and 1 ulna) treated with high energy (6000–10,000 shocks; 0.56 mJ/mm^2–0.62 mJ/mm^2 EFD). None of the atrophic nonunions[14] healed, whereas 50 of 55 (90.9%) atrophic nonunions were healed at 3 and 4 months posttreatment.[8]

Complications Complications resulting from SWT are infrequent, and when they occur, they typically require minimal, if any, treatment. None of the 631 patients reviewed by Birnbaum and colleagues[33] had a serious complication. The most common adverse effects include mild ecchymosis, petechiae, hematoma, slight swelling, and transient reddening of the skin and are usually avoidable with accurate targeting, appropriate positioning, and strict adherence to the treatment protocol.[33]

AVN

AVN is a progressive condition characterized by death of bone due to vascular insufficiency.[61] AVN primarily affects weight-bearing joints, most commonly the hip and knee.[61] Although AVN can occur in any age group, it typically occurs in a relatively young population in the third and fourth decades of their life.[61]

The precise cause of AVN remains unclear. Risk factors include trauma, surgery, steroid usage, alcoholism, coagulopathy, systemic lupus erythematosus, and lipidemia.[61]

Traditional nonoperative therapies include administration of bisphosphonates and statins, anticoagulation, and activity modification.[62] Surgical options include core decompression, vascularized and nonvascularized grafting procedures, osteotomy, and arthroplasty.[62–65] Results are variable.[15,16,63–65]

Procedure The procedure of SWT for AVN follows the same principles as discussed earlier. Because the hip is a relatively deep structure, it is important to use a high-energy technique and a relatively high number of shocks. Fluoroscopy is critical for accurate targeting.

Wang and colleagues[15,16] have reported their experience using SWT as a treatment of AVN of the femoral head. A summary of their technique is as follows:

The patient is induced with a general or regional anesthetic and positioned on a fracture table in the supine position. The affected hip is adducted and internally rotated. The location of the femoral artery is identified using digital palpation, so that the artery can be avoided during application of the shock waves. Fluoroscopy is used to identify the junctional zone between the viable and avascular bone of the femoral head. The skin overlying this junctional zone is marked with a marking pen. Ultrasound gel is applied to the skin in the area of intended treatment. The shock wave targeting device is then positioned in contact with the skin and gel. High-energy shock waves are then applied using predetermined parameters (ie, number of shocks, energy per shock, and frequency of shocks) based on the procedure and center-specific protocol.

The vital signs are monitored throughout the procedure by a member of the anesthesia team. On completion of the procedure, the groin is inspected for hematoma, swelling, and ecchymosis. The integrity of the femoral pulse and vascular status of the extremity are assessed.

Patients are transferred to the surgery recovery area where they are monitored and usually discharged later that day. Oral, nonnarcotic analgesics, such as acetaminophen, are typically recommended for any posttreatment pain. Patients are usually maintained on partial weight bearing on the affected leg for approximately 4 to 6 weeks.

Results Lin and colleagues[38] reported successful treatment of a 19-year-old patient with lupus who developed bilateral avascular necrosis of the femoral head. At 3 years' follow-up, the investigators noted that both hips had improved pain, Harris hip scores, and range of motion.[38] Imaging showed substantial reduction in bone marrow edema and no collapse of the subchondral bone.[38]

Wang and colleagues[15] compared the results of SWT with those of core decompression and bone grafting in patients with AVN of the femoral head. Patients with stage I, II, and III AVN were randomized to be treated with either high-energy SWT (single treatment, 6000 shocks, 28 kV) or core decompression and nonvascularized fibular strut grafting.[15] The groups were similar in regard to demographics, degree of pain, and function.[15]

At an average of 25 months posttreatment, the pain and Harris hip scores in the SWT group were significantly improved compared with their baseline scores, whereas the corresponding scores in the surgical group were unchanged from baseline.[15] Overall, for the SWT group, 79% of the hips were improved, 10% were unchanged, and 10% were worse.[15] Of the hips treated with a nonvascularized fibular graft, 29% were improved, 36% unchanged, and 36% worse. In the SWT group, 2 stage II and 2 stage III lesions progressed.[15] In the surgical group, 15 of the stage I or stage II lesions progressed.[15] The investigators concluded that SWT was more effective than core decompression and nonvascularized grafting in patients with early stage AVN of the femoral head.[15]

Using histopathologic and immunohistochemical techniques, the same investigators studied 14 patients (14 hips) who underwent hip arthroplasty for AVN of the femoral head.[17] Among the 14 patients, 7 received SWT before surgery, whereas the remaining did not.[17] The histopathologic examination of the femoral head revealed significantly more viable and less necrotic bone, higher cell concentration, and more cellular function in the group that received SWT.[17] The immunohistochemical analysis revealed greater concentrations of growth factors such as VEGF and von Willebrand factor, which are critical to angiogenesis, in the SWT group than the control group.[17] The investigators suggested that SWT promotes neovascularity and enhances regeneration and remodeling in avascular necrotic bone.[17]

Stress fractures

Stress fractures are overuse injuries of bone and are among the most common sports injuries. These fractures, which may be nascent or complete, result from repetitive subthreshold loading that, over time, exceeds the bone's intrinsic ability to repair itself.

Most stress fractures heal with relative rest and activity modification. Some may require a period of immobilization and protected weight bearing. High-risk stress fractures such as those involving the femoral neck, anterior cortex of the tibia, and tarsal navicular are frequently treated with surgery.[66–68] However, complications are not uncommon, and recovery is often prolonged.[66,67]

Some have proposed using low-intensity pulsed ultrasonography (LIPUS) to treat stress fractures.[55] LIPUS is safe and noninvasive.[55,69] However, as was discussed with nonunions, results have been inconsistent.[55,69] In a recent review of the literature, Busse and colleagues[69] concluded that the available evidence does not support improved healing of stress fractures treated with LIPUS.

SWT, having been shown to have a positive influence on osseous biology, has some promise as a treatment of stress fractures. SWT has several potential advantages over other forms of nonoperative treatment.

Unlike LIPUS that requires daily prolonged (up to 8–10 hours per day) use of an external coil device over the fracture site, SWT can be applied in just 1 to 2 treatment sessions.[54] The noninvasiveness of SWT makes it a particularly attractive option for individuals with open growth plates. Also, SWT can be applied safely to recalcitrant stress fractures with retained hardware that have failed surgical intervention.

At present, there are no published prospective, randomized, blinded studies that have evaluated SWT as a treatment of chronic stress fractures. That said, recent case reports have been encouraging.

Taki and colleagues[36] reported on their experience using focused SWT to treat 5 athletes with chronic stress fractures who had failed 6 to 12 months of traditional therapy. The fractures included the middle third of the tibia,[2] the base of the fifth metatarsal,[1] the inferior pubic ramus,[1] and the medial malleolus of the ankle.[1,36] A single high-energy treatment ($0.29 \, mJ/mm^2$–$0.4 \, mJ/mm^2$) was used in each case.[36] All fractures healed after SWT with time to radiographic union ranging from 2 to 3.5 months posttreatment.[36] All athletes were able to return to their sport.[36] Time to return to sport ranged from 3.5 to 6 months posttreatment.[36] There were no complications or recurrent stress fractures in any of the 5 cases.[36]

Moretti and colleagues[37] reported on 10 athletes with stress fractures of either the fifth metatarsus or tibia who received 3 to 4 sessions of low-middle energy SWT. At a mean of 8 weeks posttreatment, a 100% healing rate was noted.[37] All athletes were able to return to their preinjury level of completion.[37]

Coupled with the mechanistic studies that revealed enhanced biomechanical properties (increased bone mass and strength) and enhanced angiogenesis, these 2 case series suggest that SWT may have a role in the treatment of delayed healing of stress fractures.[18–20,27,37,38] Obviously, controlled clinical trials, ideally limited to one bone and a homogenous patient population, are necessary to confirm or refute this hypothesis.

SUMMARY

Numerous basic science and animal model studies have shown that SWT can enhance neovascularity, increase bone mass, and stimulate osteogenesis.[9,11,13,14,18–21,44,45] Clinical trials have shown that SWT can be an effective treatment of nonunions, AVN, and delayed healing of stress fractures.[3–6,33–40] The procedure is noninvasive, safe, well tolerated, easily administered, and has a high patient satisfaction rate. Recent studies have shown that SWT is as effective as surgery in some instances.[5] For these reasons, SWT should be a part of a surgeon's treatment armamentarium for these challenging clinical disorders.

REFERENCES

1. Graff J, Pastor J, Richter KD. Effect of high energy shock waves on bony tissue. Urol Res 1988;16:252–8.
2. Valchanou VD, Michailov P. High energy shock waves in the treatment of delayed and nonunion of fractures. Int Orthop 1991;15(3):181–4.
3. Schaden W, Fischer A, Sailler A. Extracorporeal shock wave therapy of nonunion or delayed osseous union. Clin Orthop Relat Res 2001;387:90–4.
4. Wang CJ, Chen HS, Chen CE, et al. Treatment of nonunions of long bone fractures with shock waves. Clin Orthop Relat Res 2001;387:95–101.
5. Cachio A, Giordano L, Colafarina O, et al. Extracorporeal shock-wave therapy compared with surgery for hypertrophic long-bone nonunions. J Bone Joint Surg 2009;91:2589–97.
6. Rompe JD, Rosendahl T, Schollner C, et al. High-energy extracorporeal shock wave treatment of nonunions. Clin Orthop Relat Res 2001;387:102–11.
7. Haupt G. Use of extracorporeal shock wave therapy in the treatment of pseudoarthrosis, tendinopathoy, and other orthopedic diseases. Urology 1997;158:4–11.
8. Xu ZH, Jiang Q, Chen DY, et al. Extracorporeal shock wave treatment in nonunions of long bone fractures. Int Orthop 2009;33:789–93.
9. Maier M, Milz S, Tischer T, et al. Influence of extracorporeal shock-wave application on normal bone in an animal model in vivo. Scintigraphy, MRI and histopathology. J Bone Joint Surg Br 2002;84(4):592–9.
10. Maier M, Averbeck B, Milz S, et al. Substance P and prostaglandin E2 release after shock wave application to the rabbit femur. Clin Orthop Relat Res 2003;406:237–45.
11. Martini L, Giavaresi G, Fini M, et al. Effect of extracorporeal shock wave therapy on osteoblastlike cells. Clin Orthop Relat Res 2003;413:269–80.
12. Johannes EJ, Kaulesar Sukul DM, Matura E. High-energy shock waves for the treatment of nonunions: an experiment on dogs. J Surg Res 1994;57(2):246–52.
13. Wang FS, Yang KD, Chen RF, et al. Extracorporeal shock wave promotes growth and differentiation of bone-marrow stromal cells towards osteoprogenitors associated with induction of TGF-beta1. J Bone Joint Surg Br 2002;84(3):457–61.
14. Wang FS, Yang KD, Kuo YR, et al. Temporal and spatial expression of bone morphogenetic proteins in extracorporeal shock wave-promoted healing of segmental defect. Bone 2003;32(4):387–96.
15. Wang CJ, Wang FS, Huang CC, et al. Treatment for osteonecrosis of the femoral head: comparison of extracorporeal shock waves with core decompression and bone-grafting. J Bone Joint Surg Am 2005;87:2380–7.
16. Wang CJ, Wang FS, Yand KD, et al. Treatment of osteonecrosis of the hip: comparison of extracorporeal shockwave with shockwave and alendronate. Arch Orthop Trauma Surg 2008;128:901–8.
17. Wang CJ, Wang FS, Ko JY, et al. Extracorporeal shockwave therapy shows regeneration in hip necrosis. Rheumatology 2008;47:542–6.
18. Wang CJ, Wang FS, Yang KD, et al. Shock wave therapy induces neovascularization at the tendon-bone junction. A study in rabbits. J Orthop Res 2003;21:984–9.
19. Wang CJ, Yang KD, Wang FS, et al. Shock wave treatment shows dose-dependent enhancement of bone mass and bone strength after fracture of the femur. Bone 2004;34:225–30.

20. Wang CJ, Wang FS, Yang KD, et al. The effect of shock wave treatment at the tendon-bone interface-an histomorphological and biomechanical study in rabbits. J Orthop Res 2005;23:274–80.

21. Wang CJ, Huang HY, Pal CH. Shock wave-enhanced neovascularisation at the tendon-bone junction: an experiment in dogs. J Foot Ankle Surg 2004;41:16–22.

22. Ma HZ, Zeng BF, Li XL. Upregulation of VEGF in subchondral bone of necrotic femoral heads in rabbits with use of extracorporeal shock waves. Calcif Tissue Int 2007;81:124–31.

23. Ma HZ, Zeng BF, Li XL, et al. Temporal and spatial expression of BMP-2 in subchondral bone of necrotic femoral heads in rabbits by use of extracorporeal shock waves. Acta Orthop 2008;79:98–105.

24. Takahashi N, Wada Y, Ohtori S, et al. Application of shock waves to rat skin decreases calcitonin gene-related peptide immunoreactivity in dorsal root ganglion neurons. Auton Neurosci 2003;107:81–4.

25. Takahashi N, Ohtori S, Saisu T, et al. Second application of low-energy shock waves has a cumulative effect on free nerve endings. Clin Orthop Relat Res 2006;443:315–9.

26. Buchbinder R, Ptasznik R, Gordon J, et al. Ultrasound-guided extracorporeal shock wave therapy for plantar fasciitis: a randomized controlled trial. JAMA 2002;288:1364–72.

27. Rompe JD, Kirkpatrick CJ, Kullmer K, et al. Dose-related effects of shock waves on rabbit tendo Achillis. A sonographic and histological study. J Bone Joint Surg Br 1998;80:546–52.

28. Sukol DM, Johannes DJ, Pierik JM, et al. The effect of high energy shock waves focused on cortical bone: an in vitro study. J Surg Res 1993;54:46–51.

29. Tischer T, Milz S, Anetzberger H, et al. [Extracorporeal shock waves induce ventral-periosteal new bone formation out of the focus zone–results of an in-vivo animal trial]. Z Orthop Ihre Grenzgeb 2002;140(3):281–5 [in German].

30. Haist J. Die Osteorestauration via Stoßwellenanwendung. Eine neue Möglichkeit zur Therapie der gestörten knöchernen Konsolidierung. In: Chaussy C, Eisenberger F, Jochum D, et al, editors. Die Stoßwelle – Forschung und Klinik. Tuebingen (Germany): Attempo; 1995. p. 157–61.

31. Ogden JA, Toth-Kischkat A, Schultheiss R. Principles of shock wave therapy. Clin Orthop Relat Res 2001;387:8–17.

32. Sems A, Dimeff R, Iannotti JP. Extracorporeal shock wave therapy in the treatment of chronic tendinopathies. J Am Acad Orthop Surg 2006;14:195–204.

33. Birnbaum K, Wirtz DC, Siebert CH, et al. Use of extracorporeal shock-wave therapy (ESWT) in the treatment of non-unions. A review of the literature. Arch Orthop Trauma Surg 2002;122(6):324–30.

34. Biedermann R, Martin A, Handle G, et al. Extracorporeal shock waves in the treatment of nonunions. J Trauma 2003;54(5):936–42.

35. Alves EM, Angrisani T, Santiago MB. The use of extracorporeal shock waves in the treatment of osteonecrosis of the femoral head: a systematic review. Clin Rheumatol 2009;28:1247–51.

36. Taki M, Iwata O, Shiono M, et al. Extracorporeal shock wave therapy for resistant stress fractures in athletes. Am J Sports Med 2007;35:1188–92.

37. Moretti B, Notarnicola A, Garofalo R, et al. Shock waves in the treatment of stress fractures. Ultrasound Med Biol 2009;35:1042–9.

38. Lin PC, Wang CJ, Yang KD, et al. Extracorporeal shockwave treatment of osteonecrosis of the femoral head in systemic lupus erythematosis. J Arthroplasty 2006;6:911–5.

39. Vogel J, Hopf C, Eysel P, et al. Application of extracorporeal shock-waves in the treatment of pseudarthrosis of the lower extremity. Preliminary results. Arch Orthop Trauma Surg 1997;116(8):480–3.

40. Petrisor BA, Lisson S, Sprague S. Extracorporeal shockwave therapy: a systematic review of its use in fracture management. Indian J Orthop 2009;43:161–7.

41. Schleberger R, Delius M, Dahmen GP. Orthopedic extracorporeal shock wave therapy (ESWT): method anaylsis and suggestion of a prospective study design-consensus report. In: Chaussy C, Eisenberger F, Jocham D, et al, editors. High energy shock waves in medicine. Stuttgart (Germany): Thieme; 1997. p. 108–11.

42. Gerdesmeyer L, Henne M, Gobel M, et al. Physical principles and generation of shockwaves. In: Gerdsmeyer L, editor. Extracorporeal shock wave therapy: technologies, basics, clinical results. Towson (MD): Data Trace Media; 2007. p. 11–20.

43. Lohrer H, Natuck T, Dorn-Lange NV, et al. Comparison of radial versus focused extracorporeal shock waves in plantar fasciitis using functional measures. Foot Ankle Int 2010;31:1–9.

44. Martini L, Fini M, Giavaresi G, et al. Primary osteoblasts response to shock wave therapy using different parameters. Artif Cells Blood Substit Immobil Biotechnol Nov 2003;31(4):449–66.

45. Maier M, Hausdorf J, Tischer T, et al. [New bone formation by extracorporeal shock waves. Dependence of induction on energy flux density]. Orthopade 2004;33(12):1401–10 [in German].

46. Rompe JD, Meurer A, Nafe B, et al. Repetitive low-energy shock wave application without local anesthesia is more efficient than repetitive low-energy shock wave application with local anesthesia in the treatment of chronic plantar fasciitis. J Orthop Res 2005;23:931–41.

47. Labek G, Auersperg V, Ziernhold M, et al. Influence of local anesthesia and energy level on the clinical outcome of extracorporeal shock wave-treatment of chronic plantar fasciitis. Z Orthop Ihre Grenzgeb 2005;143:240–6.

48. LaVelle DG. Delayed union and nonunion of fractures. In: Canale TS, editor. Campbell's operative orthopaedics. 9th edition. St Louis (MO): Mosby; 1998. p. 2579–629.

49. Rosenberg GA, Sferra JJ. Treatment strategies for acute fractures and nonunions of the proximal fifth metatarsal. J Am Acad Orthop Surg 2000;8(5):332–8.

50. Torg JS, Balduini FC, Zelco RR, et al. Fractures of the base of the fifth metatarsal distal to the tuberosity: classification and guidelines for non-surgical and surgical management. J Bone Joint Surg Am 1984;66:209–14.

51. Kavanaugh JH, Brower TD, Mann RV. The Jones fracture revisited. J Bone Joint Surg Am 1970;60:776–82.

52. Dameron TB Jr. Fractures of the proximal fifth metatarsal: selecting the best treatment option. J Am Acad Orthop Surg 1995;3(2):110–4.

53. Wright RW, Fischer DA, Shively RA, et al. Refracture of proximal fifth metatarsal fractures after intramedullary screw fixation in athletes. Am J Sports Med 2000; 28(5):732–6.

54. Holmes GB Jr. Treatment of delayed unions and nonunions of the proximal fifth metatarsal with pulsed electromagnetic fields. Foot Ankle Int 1994;15(10):552–6.

55. Brand JC, Brindle T, Nyland J. Does pulsed low intensity ultrasound allow early return to normal activities when treating stress fractures? Iowa Orthop J 1999; 19:26–30.

56. Saltzman C, Lightfoot A, Amendola A. PEMF as treatment for delayed healing of foot and ankle arthrodesis. Foot Ankle Int 2004;25(11):771–3.

57. Foley KT, Mroz TE, Arnold PM, et al. Randomized, prospective, and controlled clinical trial of pulsed electromagnetic field stimulation for cervical fusion. Spine J 2008;8(3):436–42.

58. Heckman JD. Rockwood and Green's fractures in adults. 5th edition. Philadelphia: Lippincott Williams and Wilkins; 2001.

59. Warren SB, Brooker AF. Intramedullary nailing of tibial nonunions. Clin Orthop 1992;285:236–43.

60. Younger EM, Chapman MW. Morbidity at bone graft donor sites. J Orthop Trauma 1989;3:192–5.

61. Malizos KN, Karantanas AH, Vartimidis SE, et al. Osteonecrosis of the femoral head: etiology, imaging, and treatment. Eur J Radiol 2007;63:16–28.

62. Parsons JS, Stelle N. Osteonecrosis of the femoral head: part 2-options for treatment. Curr Orthop 2008;22:349–58.

63. Koo KH, Kim R, Ko GH, et al. Preventing collapse in early osteonecrosis of the femoral head. A randomised clinical trial of core decompression. J Bone Joint Surg Br 1995;77:870–4.

64. Learmonth ID, Maloon S, Dall G. Core decompression for early atraumatic osteonecrosis of the femoral head. J Bone Joint Surg Br 1990;72:387–90.

65. Salto S, Ohzono K, Ono K. Joint-preserving operations for idiopathic avascular necrosis of the femoral head. Results of core decompression, grafting, and osteotomy. J Bone Joint Surg Am 1988;70:78–84.

66. Chang PS, Harris RM. Intramedullary nailing for chronic tibial stress fractures. A review of five cases. Am J Sports Med 1996;24:688–92.

67. DeLee JC, Evans JP, Julian J. Stress fracture of the fifth metatarsal. Am J Sports Med 1983;11:349–53.

68. Varner KE, Younas SA, Lintner DM, et al. Chronic anterior midtibial stress fractures in athletes treated with reamed intramedullary nailing. Am J Sports Med 2005;33:1071–6.

69. Busse JW, Kaur J, Mollon B, et al. Low intensity pulsed ultrasonography for fractures: systematic review of randomised controlled trials. Low intensity pulsed ultrasonography for fractures: systematic review of randomised controlled trials. BMJ 2009;338:b11.

Bone Block Lengthening of the Proximal Interphalangeal Joint for Managing the Floppy Toe Deformity

Mark S. Myerson, MD[a],*, Jorge Filippi, MD[b]

KEYWORDS

• Floppy toe • Graft • Arthrodesis • Deformity

The short floppy toe, an iatrogenic condition in which the digit lacks structural stability, results from excessive resection of the distal aspect of the proximal phalanx during correction of claw or hammer toe deformity.[1–5] In 1979, Newman and Fitton[6] reported a short and flail toe in 23% of patients who had undergone proximal interphalangeal (PIP) resection arthroplasty, but the overall rate of flail toe after PIP arthroplasty has not been reported in the literature. Although the authors generally remove about 4 mm of the distal portion of the proximal phalanx during arthroplasty, the exact amount of bone resection that leads to a short and floppy toe has not been described. Patients with floppy toe complain of pain from shoe irritation and instability with catching of the toes on shoes, socks, or stockings and invariably hate the appearance of the toe. Patients lack voluntary motion in the toe and have multidirectional instability at the PIP joint. The involved toe is much shorter than the adjacent digit, which it will often overlap. In addition to the PIP joint, it is important to evaluate the metatarsophalangeal (MP) joint, which may also be quite unstable (**Fig. 1**). It is not uncommon for a patient with a short floppy toe to present with an overlapping digit, the result of a crossover toe deformity, which was never correctly straightened at the MP joint. Needless to state, if one approaches the correction of a crossover toe deformity as if it were a hammer or claw toe, then recurrent deformity is likely, even if the toe is now out to length. It is important to establish the circulation to the toe preoperatively. Any lengthening may cause ischemia to the toe, and it is helpful to assess this and the presence of any

[a] Institute for Foot and Ankle Reconstruction, Mercy Medical Center, 301 St Paul Place, Baltimore MD 21202, USA
[b] Department of Orthopedic Surgery, Pontifical Catholic University of Chile, Marcoleta 352 Patio Interior, Santiago 833-0033, Chile
* Corresponding author.
E-mail address: mark4feet@aol.com

Foot Ankle Clin N Am 15 (2010) 663–668
doi:10.1016/j.fcl.2010.09.001
1083-7515/10/$ – see front matter © 2010 Elsevier Inc. All rights reserved.

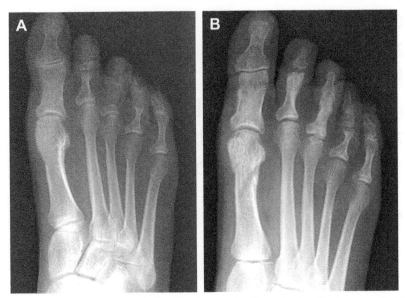

Fig. 1. The third toe was extremely short and unstable after prior forefoot surgery. Excessive bone had been removed form the proximal phalanx of the third toe. The second toe PIP joint was also unstable and painful, although not short (*A*). These deformities were corrected with a lengthening bone block allograft arthrodesis of the third toe PIP joint and a revision with arthrodesis of the second toe interphalangeal joint (*B*).

underlying diseases, particularly diabetes, before reconstruction. The radiographs always demonstrate the extent of the shortening and deformity, and this finding is taken into consideration when planning correction.

SURGICAL TREATMENT

The flail toe can be corrected surgically by lengthening and/or stabilizing the toe. Several procedures have been described for the correction of the flail toe, including syndactylization to an adjacent toe,[7] free autologous bone graft arthrodesis of the PIP joint,[3–5] transposition of an osteocutaneous flap from the hallux to the second toe,[8] and the use of external fixator for gradual lengthening.[2] Also, partial or total amputation of the toe[9] could be considered in elderly patients or those with underlying vascular disease (**Fig. 2**).

Syndactylization is a poor operative choice because it worsens the cosmesis, does not correct the length of the toe, and rarely improves the stability of either digit, frequently pulling the previously normal digit into extension; thus, continued instability remains a problem. The hemipulp osteocutaneous island flap, procured from the lateral one-third of the distal phalanx of the hallux, was described by Koshima and colleagues.[8] This technique has some disadvantages caused by the technical difficulty, the alteration of the appearance of the hallux, and the limitation of the second toe because of the limited movement of the flap. In 2009, Lamm and Ades[2] described in a patient with Raynaud disease, a 2 -stage approach involving gradual lengthening with external fixator and the use of autologous bone graft with good results. The total time to correct the deformity with external fixator was 15 weeks. In 1992, Mahan[3] described an arthrodesis technique for lengthening the toe using autogenous calcaneal graft at the PIP joint for correcting flail toe in one patient. The authors' preferred

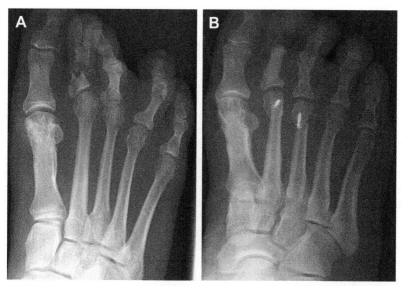

Fig. 2. Radiograph of the foot of a patient who had undergone multiple prior surgeries, first with correction of hallux valgus with a distal first metatarsal osteotomy and marked shortening of the first metatarsal. This correction was followed by toe surgery, with further complications because the crossover toe at the second and third MP joints were not addressed, excessive bone was removed from the second toe PIP joint, and the toe was left short and floppy (A). A shortening osteotomy of the distal second and third metatarsals, and an allograft lengthening arthrodesis of the second PIP joint were performed, with good alignment and bone healing at 10 weeks after surgery and removal of the Kirschner wire (B).

management for the correction of the short and floppy toe is the technique using a structural bone block graft, performed in one stage, to restore the length, stability, function, and appearance of the digit.[10]

SURGICAL TECHNIQUE

The procedure is performed with a dorsal longitudinal incision extending from the MP joint to the middle phalanx. During the dissection of the soft tissues, the extensor hood and extensor tendons are carefully preserved, although a lengthening of the extensor tendons is commonly required. Tendon lengthening is not always necessary because as the toe is lengthened, the more normal tension on the extensor apparatus is restored, but this decision depends on the presence of a contracture at the MP joint. Correction of both the interphalangeal and the MP joint deformity is necessary for most patients and is performed with a soft tissue release at the level of the MP joint, with capsulotomy, collateral ligament release, or tendon lengthening as required. Shortening osteotomies of the metatarsals may also be necessary, particularly if there is a long metatarsal associated with a crossover toe. The interphalangeal joint is then exposed, including the base of the middle phalanx and the remnant of the distal portion of the proximal phalanx. A 2-mm burr is then used with cold irrigation to prepare the bone surfaces for arthrodesis. The base of the middle phalanx is preserved removing only the articular cartilage, and the distal portion of the proximal phalanx is debrided to the bleeding bone. There is often a thick fibrous cap over the distal portion of the remaining proximal phalanx, which must be removed to obtain an arthrodesis.

The bone graft may be harvested from either the ipsilateral calcaneus or from a piece of iliac crest autograft or allograft. In each case, the graft must be structural, with cortical bone on 2 of its surfaces for maximum support. In general, the authors place one of the cortical surfaces dorsally and then mix the graft with concentrated bone marrow aspirate from the iliac crest. The length of the graft is established by the desired length of the toe, which is ascertained by inserting a small laminar spreader between the proximal and middle phalanges. The surgery is not performed with any tourniquet to guarantee that the toe has circulation with maximum elongation. It is quite easy to visualize when the toe is too long, and if ischemia occurs, the graft has to be shortened slightly. Furthermore, when the Kirschner (K) wire is inserted further, slight ischemia develops, and this too must be taken into consideration if the toe is poorly perfused. The graft is then contoured to shape, with the length determined by the desired length of the toe and the width and depth by the shape of the phalanges. It is preferable to contour the graft slightly such that a cup-and-cone fit is present on the distal bone surfaces, although this fit depends on the geometry of the remnant of the phalanges. In general, after debridement with the burr, the middle phalanx presents a cup shape to the graft and the distal part of the proximal phalanx a cone shape, which is then matched with the reciprocal shape of the graft. Once the graft is cut to the desired shape and size, it is cannulated with a 1.2-mm smooth K wire. This hole facilitates the insertion of the final K wire and prevents spinning of the graft once the K wire enters the graft in the toe. A similar sized K-wire hole is then made through the middle phalanx antegrade out the toe. A threaded K wire is used because a smooth pin will loosen with time and these pins need to be left in for at least 8 weeks when arthrodesis may be present. Following the use of the smaller K wire for the pilot hole preparation in the graft and distal phalanges, a slightly larger (1.6 mm) threaded K wire is introduced through the pilot hole in the middle phalanx, antegrade out of the toe and then retrograde into the bone graft (**Fig. 3**). Because this is a threaded K wire, the graft must be firmly held and compressed against the

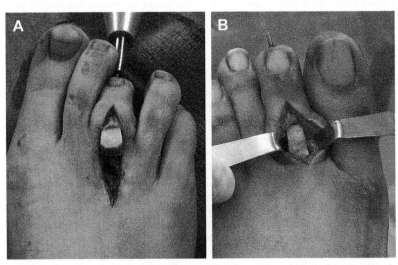

Fig. 3. The bone graft in situ after insertion and fixation with a threaded 1.6-mm K wire (A). The graft has been inserted in a different foot and secured with fixation into the base of the proximal phalanx (B).

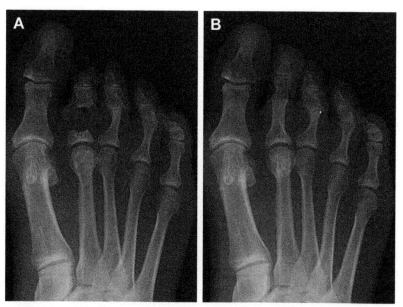

Fig. 4. Insertion and fixation of a graft in this foot is difficult because of the very small size of the base of the proximal phalanx that is left (*A*). To secure and fix the graft in place, the K wire has to be very slightly angled into the proximal corner of the base of the phalanx. The radiograph shows that the graft has healed well 1 year after surgery (*B*).

middle phalanx while the wire is introduced. The toe is then distracted by pulling on the distal phalanx, and with the graft now attached to the middle phalanx, the toe is levered into position and the wire introduced into the base of the proximal phalanx. The wire should not cross the MP joint because it is left in place for a long time and this threaded pin will easily break. The patient is permitted to bear weight immediately in a protective surgical shoe as determined by comfort. The wire is left in place until an arthrodesis is present on radiographs or until a complication such as an infection occurs (**Fig. 4**).

SUMMARY

Little attention has been given to the cause and treatment of the floppy toe deformity in the literature. As an iatrogenic condition, the best treatment is prevention. Although the amount of resection of the proximal phalanx necessary to develop a flail toe after fixed hammer toe repair is not described, it is recommended to resect only the supracondylar aspect of the proximal phalanx[11] to avoid later instability. Initial treatment of this condition includes taping, padding, splinting, or the use of orthotic arch supports. Surgical correction of this deformity is challenging because it requires a careful balance of the bone and tendon lengths to give support to the toe. The prior scarring and deformity with the potential for ischemic complications add to the difficulty of the surgery, and amputation of the toe may have to be an alternative in low-demand patients, elderly patients, or patients with underlying vascular disease. A structural bone block graft lengthening for correction of the short floppy toe deformity has been proved to be effective in providing stability and improving cosmesis for most patients.

REFERENCES

1. Coughlin MJ. Lesser toe abnormalities. J Bone Joint Surg Am 2002;84:1446–69.
2. Lamm BM, Ades JK. Gradual digital lengthening with autologous bone graft and external fixation for correction of flail toe in a patient with Raynaud's disease. J Foot Ankle Surg 2009;48:488–94.
3. Mahan KT. Bone graft reconstruction of a flail digit. J Am Podiatr Med Assoc 1992;82:264–8.
4. Mahan KT, Downey MS, Weinfeld GD. Autogenous bone graft interpositional arthrodesis for the correction of flail toe: a retrospective analysis of 22 procedures. J Am Podiatr Med Assoc 2003;93:167–73.
5. Myerson MS. "Correction of lesser toe deformity". In: Myerson MS, editor. Reconstructive foot and ankle surgery. Philadelphia: Elsevier Saunders; 2005. p. 98–9.
6. Newman RJ, Fitton JM. An evaluation of operative procedures in the treatment of hammertoe. Acta Orthop Scand 1979;50:709–12.
7. Marek L, Giacopelli J, Granoff D. Syndactylization for the treatment of fifth toe deformities. J Am Podiatr Med Assoc 1991;81:248–52.
8. Koshima I, Shozia M, Soeda S. Osteocutaneous flap from the big toe for repair of osteomyelitis of the second toe. Ann Plast Surg 1990;25:283–6.
9. Gallentine JW, DeOrio JK. Removal of the second toe for severe hammertoe deformity in elderly patients. Foot Ankle Int 2005;26:353–8.
10. Myerson MS, Filippi J. Interphalangeal joint lengthening arthrodesis for the treatment of the flail toe. Foot Ankle Int, in press.
11. Coughlin MJ. Operative repair of fixed hammertoe deformity. Foot Ankle Int 2000; 21:94–104.

Index

Note: Page numbers of article titles are in **boldface** type.

A

Adjunctive treatments, with bone grafting, biologics as, **577–596**. See also
   Bone morphogenetic proteins (BMPs).
         poor bone healing risk and, relative need based on, 647
         cost considerations of, 589–591, 605
         growth factors as, **597–609**. See also *Growth factors.*
         in foot and ankle procedures, 578–579, 583, 585, 588–589
Age factor, of mesenchymal stem cell grafts, 613
Agility total ankle replacement, platelet-rich plasma for, 644–645
Allografts, of bone, allograft stem cells combined with, 611–614
         chips for backfilling, in proximal tibial autologous graft harvest, 556
         pros and cons of, 559
         surgical incorporation of, 545, 577
         with intramedullary nail fixation, 546
   of stem cells, allograft bone combined with, 611–614
α-BSM (bone substitute material), 568
American Orthopaedic Foot and Ankle Society (AOFAS), Ankle-Hindfoot Scale of, in
   recombinant human platelet-derived growth factor clinical trials, 634
Angiogenesis, in bone formation, 624, 626–627, 629
         shock wave therapy impact on, 653–654
         tissue, following injury, 612
Ankle arthrodeses, bone morphogenetic proteins for, 578
         recombinant human BMP-2 studies of, 545–546, 578–579, 583–585
               average time to healing, 583
               case presentation of, 586, 589–591
               case presentation of foot vs., 587–588, 592–594
               case presentation of tibia vs., 586–588
               comorbidities and, 595
               complications of, 592–593
               cost considerations of, 589–591
               determination of time to healing, 583
               discussion on, 588–595
               further research on, 595
               material and methods for, 578–579
               osteoconductor indications with, 594–595
               overall results vs., 579
               patient categorization for, 579
               patient database of, 580–585
               patient risk level and, 593
               salvage procedures and, 593–594
               segmental tibial bone loss example vs., 583, 585, 601

Foot Ankle Clin N Am 15 (2010) 669–687
doi:10.1016/S1083-7515(10)00082-3
1083-7515/10/$ – see front matter © 2010 Elsevier Inc. All rights reserved.

foot.theclinics.com

Ankle arthrodeses (*continued*)
        sponge application technique in, 591–592
        subtalar fusion example vs., 583, 585, 593
        talonavicular fusion example vs., 583–584
        used alone vs. with adjuncts, 583, 585
    recombinant human platelet-derived growth factor for, **621–640**. See also
        Augment Bone Graft.
Ankle fractures, osteoporotic, calcium sulfate grafts for, 563–567
Antibiotics, calcium sulfate graft indications for, 563
Arthritis, end-stage foot and ankle, arthrodeses for, 621
        autogenous bone graft used with, 621–622
        platelet-derived growth factor used with, 622–636. See also
            Recombinant human platelet-derived growth factor (rhPDGF-BB).
Arthrodeses. See also *Fusion.*
    bone morphogenetic proteins for, 578
        retrospective review of, 545–546, 578
    of ankle. See *Ankle arthrodeses.*
    of foot. See *Foot arthrodeses.*
    of proximal interphalangeal joint, for flail toe correction, 664–666
        tibial bone grafts for, 554–557. See also *Tibial bone grafts.*
        tissue engineering for, 544
Arthroplasty, resection, of proximal interphalangeal joint, for floppy toe deformity, 663–665
Augment Bone Graft, for foot and ankle fusion, discussion on, 635–636
        prospective 60-patient open-label Canadian registration trial on, 631–632
        prospective 434-patient North American pivotal trial on, 634–635
        prospective randomized controlled 20-patient US pilot trial on, 632–634
Autogenous grafts, of bone. See *Autologous bone grafts/grafting (ABG).*
Autografts, of bone. See *Autologous bone grafts/grafting (ABG).*
Autoimmune response, mesenchymal stem cell grafts and, 612
Autologous bone grafts/grafting (ABG), for foot and ankle procedures, as gold
    standard, 559, 577, 597
        bone morphogenetic proteins used with, 578–579, 589. See also
            Recombinant human BMP-2 (rhBMP-2).
        in adverse scenarios, 601–605
    cost considerations of, 605
    donor site proximity to surgical site, 554
    for end-stage arthritis, 621–622
        platelet-derived growth factor used with, 622–636. See also *Recombinant human*
            platelet-derived growth factor (rhPDGF-BB).
    free, for flail toe correction, 664
    growth factors added to, **597–609**. See also *Growth factors.*
    harvesting of, 559
    iliac crest grafts in. See *Autologous iliac crest bone graft (AICBG).*
    limitations of, 577–578, 603
    problems with, 559
    summary overview of, 557
    surgical incorporation of, 545, 577
    tibial bone grafts in, **553–558**. See also *Tibial bone grafts.*
    with intramedullary nail fixation, 546–547
        adjunctive treatments for, 598–601
    for spinal fusion, 603–604

Autologous iliac crest bone graft (AICBG), bone marrow aspiration technique
    for, 615–616
    for foot and ankle procedures, 553–554
        advantages of, 553–554
        complications of, 554, 597–598
        tibial fracture union rates with, 598–600
        tibial grafts vs., 554
    for fracture nonunion, in adverse scenarios, 601–605
        limitations of, 603–604
        success rates with, 598–600, 603
    in floppy toe surgery, 666
Avascular necrosis (AVN), description of, 656
    shock wave therapy for, procedure for, 656–657
        results of, 657
        trends of, 651–652, 656
    stem cell grafting for, 611

B

Backfilling, in proximal tibial autologous graft harvest, 555–556
Basic fibroblast growth factor (FGF2), bone healing function of, 642
β-Tricalcium phosphate (β-TCP)/collagen, as bone substitute material, bone marrow
    aspiration technique for, 615–617
        FDA approval of, 614
        graft processing steps for, 616–617
        granules of, 570
            recombinant human platelet-derived growth factor combined with, 622–623,
                629–630
        mesenchymal stem cell grafts vs., 611–615
        with concentrated bone marrow aspirate, 614–615
Bibbo host-surgical site classification system, to assess bone-healing risk, 646–647
        relative osteobiologic adjuvant need based on, 647
Bioabsorbable ceramics, as scaffolds, 560
Bioactive ceramics, as scaffolds, 560
Bioinert ceramics, as scaffolds, 560
Biologic response modifiers, 598
Biology/biologics, for fracture manipulation, advances in, 544–545
        shock wave therapy as, **651–662**. See also *Shock wave therapy (SWT)*.
    in foot and ankle surgery, **577–596**. See also *Recombinant human BMP-2 (rhBMP-2)*.
        strategic development of, 598
    in tissue engineering, 543–544
        bone morphogenetic proteins and, 543–547, 598. See also *Bone morphogenetic*
        proteins (BMPs).
Biomet trocar, for bone marrow harvest between iliac walls, 615–616
Blood clot stabilization, in bone formation, 623–625
BMP-7 Italian Observational Study (BIOS) Group, 601–602
Bone block lengthening, of proximal interphalangeal joint, for floppy toe deformity, **663–668**
        description of, 663–664
        summary overview of, 667
        surgical technique for, 665–667
        surgical treatment alternatives vs., 664–665

Bone chips, allograft, for backfilling, in proximal tibial autologous graft harvest, 556
Bone formation, biologic stimuli for, 544–545, 611
    bone morphogenetic proteins role in, 601. See also *Bone morphogenetic*
        proteins (BMPs).
    cellular requirements for, 544
        growth/differentiation factor inducement of, 548–549
    mesenchymal stem cells role in, 612, 623–624
    new, 545
    periosteal, shock wave therapy impact on, 654
    platelet-derived growth factor role of, 623–625
    synthetic bone grafts and, 560
Bone fusion, physiological. See *Bone healing*.
    surgical. See *Arthrodeses; Fusion*.
Bone grafts/grafting, autografts vs. allografts, 559, 577. See also *Allografts;*
    Autologous bone grafts/grafting (ABG).
        surgical incorporation of, 545
        with intramedullary nail fixation, 546–547
    clinical indications for, 559
    donor vs. recipient site locations of, 554
    harvest of. See *Graft harvest*.
    in floppy toe surgery, harvesting of, 666
        insertion and fixation of, 666–667
    limitations of, 635–636
    mesenchymal stem cells for, **611–619**
        advances in, 611
        as allograft, 612–613
        beta-tricalcium phosphate/collagen vs., 614–617
        culture-expanded, 612
        handling of graft, 612–613
        in humans, 612
        rationale for, 613
        suitable usage of, 614
        summary overview of, 618
        Trinity Evolution allograft and, 611–612
        xenograft source of, 612
    osteoconductive properties of, 544, 553
    osteoinductive properties of, 544–545, 553
    platelet-rich plasma for augmentation of, **641–649**. See also *Platelet-rich plasma (PRP)*.
        practical clinical considerations for, 647–648
    recombinant human platelet-derived growth factor and, **621–640**. See also
        Recombinant human platelet-derived growth factor (rhPDGF-BB).
    substitutes for. See *Bone substitute material (BSM)*.
    synthetic, **559–576**. See also *Synthetic bone grafts/grafting*.
    tibial, **553–558**. See also *Tibial bone grafts*.
    with intramedullary nail fixation, 546–547
        bone morphogenetic proteins and, 546–547, 578
Bone healing, bone morphogenetic proteins impact on, in foot and ankle surgery, 577–578.
    See also *Recombinant human BMP-2 (rhBMP-2)*.
        retrospective review of, 545–546, 578
    cascade of events leading to, 577, 612, 624–625
    orthobiologic agents for, 545, 560, 612

host-surgical site indications for, 647
   risks for poor, 641–642
      Bibbo classification system for, 646–647
      relative osteobiologic adjuvant need based on, 647
Bone loss. See *Segmental bone loss.*
Bone marrow aspiration (BMA), concentrated, β-tricalcium phosphate/collagen with, 614–615
   surgical technique for, 615–617
Bone matrix/matrices, for mesenchymal stem cell grafts, 613
   in bone formation, 624
   in tissue engineering, 544, 548
   synthetic grafts and, 560, 570–571
Bone mineral density (BMD), shock wave therapy impact on, 653–654
Bone morphogenetic proteins (BMPs), **543–551**
   for surgical tissue engineering, 543–547
      advances in, 543–544
      autologous bone grafts used with, 578–579, 598
         in adverse scenarios, 601–605
      clinical indications and outcomes in, 544
         recent studies of, 545–546
         retrospective review of, 545–546
      complications associated with, 547
      cost considerations of, 589–591, 605
      definitions in, 543–544, 577
      electrospinning and, 547
      fixation devices and, 545
      future trends for, 547–549
      in foot and ankle surgery, 577–578. See also *Recombinant human BMP-2 (rhBMP-2); Recombinant human BMP-7 (rhBMP-7).*
      in fracture care, 546
         for nonunion repair, 546–547
         initial experimental work on, 599–601
      in soft tissue repair, 548–549
      initial description of, 545
      mechanism of action, 545
      methods for incorporation of, 545
      natural healing process vs., 544
      observational studies of, 601–603
      osteoconduction and, 544
      osteoinduction and, 544–545
      percutaneous administration of, 604
      polylactic-co-glycolic acid vs., 547–548
      polyphosphazene polymers vs., 547
      prospective studies of, 635
      shock wave therapy impact on, 653
      summary overview of, 549
      tendon repair and, 548–549
   sequential expression of, in bone formation, 625–626
Bone repair process. See *Bone healing.*
Bone Source cement, 566
Bone substitute material (BSM), α-BSM, 568

β-tricalcium phosphate as, bone marrow aspiration technique for, 615–617
     FDA approval of, 614
     graft processing steps for, 616–617
     granules of, 570
          recombinant human platelet-derived growth factor combined with, 622–623, 629–630
     mesenchymal stem cell grafts vs., 611–614
     with concentrated bone marrow aspirate, 614–615
  chemistry of, 560
  in tissue engineering, 544
  marketing of, 560
  surgical incorporation of, 545
     bone morphogenetic proteins and, 547–548, 600
  synthetic, **559–576.** See also *Synthetic bone grafts/grafting.*
Bone transfer, docking site during, graft expansion consideration of, 604–605
Bone-tendon junctions, shock wave therapy impact on, 653

C

Calcaneal fractures, displaced intraarticular, calcium phosphate grafts for, 567–568
Calcium phosphate, as synthetic bone grafts, 560, 563–568
     plus calcium sulfate, 569
     plus osteoinductive matrix, 570–571
     plus recombinant human bone morphogenetic protein plus polymers as, 571
Calcium sulfate, as synthetic bone grafts, 560–563
     plus calcium phosphate, 569
Calcium-based ceramics, for backfilling, in proximal tibial autologous graft harvest, 556
     osteoconductive properties of, 544, 560
Callus formation, in bone repair process, 624
Canadian registration trial, prospective 60-patient open-label, on recombinant human platelet-derived growth factor, 631–632
          discussion on, 635–636
Cellular proliferation, in bone formation, 625
Centrifuge, of bone marrow aspiration, 616
Ceramics, as scaffolds, categories of, 560
     calcium-based, for backfilling, in proximal tibial autologous graft harvest, 556
     osteoconductive properties of, 544, 560
Charcot neuroarthropathy, recombinant human BMP-2 and, 595
Chemistry, in tissue engineering, 543–544
     of bone graft substitutes, 560. See also *Synthetic bone grafts/grafting.*
Chemotaxis, cellular, in bone formation, 625–627
Claw toe, floppy toe deformity and, 663
Clinical focusing, for shock wave therapy, 654
Clinical trials, on recombinant human platelet-derived growth factor, for foot and ankle fusion, discussion on, 635–636
          prospective 60-patient open-label Canadian registration, 631–632
          prospective 434-patient North American pivotal, 634–635
          prospective randomized controlled 20-patient US pilot, 632–634
Collagen, for bone grafting, 614–615. See also *β-Tricalcium phosphate (β-TCP)/collagen.*
     osteoconductive properties of, 544, 611
     synthesis of, growth/differentiation factor inducement of, 548–549

Comorbidities, in foot and ankle surgery, recombinant human BMP-2 use and, 595
Composite synthetic bone grafts, 569–571
    calcium phosphate plus osteoinductive matrix as, 570–571
    calcium phosphate recombinant human bone morphogenetic protein plus polymers
        as, 571
    calcium sulfate plus calcium phosphate as, 569–570
Cost of adjunctive treatments, for bone grafting, in foot and ankle procedures,
    589–591, 605
Crossover toe deformity, floppy toe deformity and, 663, 665
Culture-expanded mesenchymal stem cells, 612
Curettes, for tibial autologous graft harvest, 555, 557
Cytokines, immunomodulatory, in injured tissue, 612–613

D

Delayed union, of fractures, bone morphogenetic proteins for, 578
        shock wave therapy for, 651–652, 657–658
        tissue engineering for, 544
Dimethyl sulfoxide (DMSO) cryoprotectant, for Trinity Evolution allograft, 612
Distal tibial bone grafts, for foot and ankle procedures, 556–557
        authors' preferred harvest technique for, 557
    medial incision for harvest of, 557
Distraction osteogenesis, graft expansion consideration of, 604–605
    recombinant human platelet-derived growth factor for, 630
Docking site, during bone transfer, graft expansion consideration of, 604–605
Donor sites. See also *Graft harvest.*
    for autologous bone grafting, in foot and ankle procedures, 554
Drill, for tibial autologous graft harvest, 555, 557

E

Efficacy, of recombinant human BMP-7, 601–603
    of recombinant human platelet-derived growth factor, 635–636
Electricity, tissue engineering and, 544
Electrospinning, for bone healing materials, bone morphogenetic proteins and, 547–549
End-stage arthritis, of foot and ankle, arthrodeses for, 621
        autogenous bone graft used with, 621–622
        platelet-derived growth factor used with, 622–636. See also *Recombinant human
        platelet-derived growth factor (rhPDGF-BB).*
Energy flux density (EFD), in shock wave therapy, 653–654
Engineering principles, in tissue engineering, 543–544
Epidermal growth factor (EGF), bone healing function of, 642
External fixation, tissue engineering and, 545

F

Fibroblast growth factor (FGF2), basic, bone healing function of, 642
Fibroblasts, platelet-derived growth factors expression by, 623
Fixation devices and techniques, for calcaneal fractures, calcium phosphate grafts for,
    567–568
    for spinal fusion, 603–604

Fixation (*continued*)
    for tibial fractures, intramedullary nail fixation as, autologous bone grafts with, 598–600
        bone morphogenetic proteins used with, 546–547, 578, 601
    in floppy toe surgery, 665–667
    of osteoporotic ankle fractures, calcium sulfate grafts for, 563–567
    tissue engineering and, 544–545
Flail toe, description of, 663–664
    surgical management of, **663–668**. See also *Bone block lengthening*.
Floppy toe deformity, bone block lengthening of proximal interphalangeal joint for, **663–668**
    description of, 663–664
    summary overview of, 667
    surgical technique for, 665–667
    surgical treatment alternatives vs., 664–665
Foot arthrodeses, bone morphogenetic proteins for, recombinant human BMP-2 studies of,
    579, 583–585
        average time to healing, 583
        case presentation of, 587–588, 592–594
        case presentation of ankle vs., 586, 589–591
        case presentation of tibia vs., 586–588
        comorbidities and, 595
        complications of, 592–593
        cost considerations of, 589–591
        determination of time to healing, 583
        discussion on, 588–595
        further research on, 595
        material and methods for, 578–579
        osteoconductor indications with, 594–595
        overall results vs., 579
        patient categorization for, 579
        patient database of, 580–585
        patient risk level and, 593
        salvage procedures and, 593–594
        segmental tibial bone loss example vs., 583, 585, 601
        sponge application technique in, 591–592
        subtalar fusion example vs., 583, 585, 593
        talonavicular fusion example vs., 583–584
        used alone vs. with adjuncts, 583, 585
    recombinant human platelet-derived growth factor for, **621–640**. See also *Augment*
        Bone Graft.
Fractures, ankle, osteoporotic, calcium sulfate grafts for, 563–567
    bone morphogenetic proteins for. See also *Recombinant human BMP-2 (rhBMP-2)*;
        Recombinant human BMP-7 (rhBMP-7).
        in long bones, 546–547, 604
        tibial studies of, 546–547, 578
    calcaneal, calcium phosphate grafts for, 567–568
    delayed union of. See *Delayed union*.
    following tibial bone grafting in foot and ankle arthrodesis, 555, 557
    lower extremity, tibial bone grafts for, distal, 556–557
        proximal, 554–556
    nonunion of. See *Nonunion*.
    platelet-rich plasma in treatment of, 643

recombinant human platelet-derived growth factor for, 630
stress, following tibial bone grafting in foot and ankle arthrodesis, 557
    shock wave therapy for, 651, 657–658
tibial. See *Tibial fractures.*
tissue engineering for, 544, 611–612
Fusion. See also *Arthrodeses.*
    spinal (lumbar), autologous iliac crest bone graft for, 603–604
        recombinant human BMP-7 used in, 602–603
    subtalar, recombinant human BMP-2 used in, 583, 585, 593
    talonavicular, recombinant human BMP-2 used in, 583–584

G

GEM 21S, as recombinant human platelet-derived growth factor, 629–630
Gene technology, recombinant, for manufacturing osteoinductive proteins, 578, 599–600
Graft harvest, of bone grafts, autologous, 559, 597–598
    for floppy toe surgery, 666
    of iliac crest bone. See *Autologous iliac crest bone graft (AICBG).*
    of mesenchymal stem cells, 613
    of tibial bone grafts, distal, 557
        proximal, 555–556
Granulation, in bone formation, 624
Growth factors, in platelet-rich plasma, bone healing function of, 641–643
    concentrating system for, 647
    shock wave therapy impact on, 653
    tissue engineering and, 544–545
    with autologous bone grafts, **546–609**
        advanced strategies for, 597–598
        fracture union rates observed in, 601–602
        in adverse scenarios, 604–605
        reaming by-products vs., 598–600, 604
        tibial fracture union rates and, with growth factors, 599–603
            without growth factors, 598–600
Growth/differentiation factors (GDFs), for tendon repair, 548–549

H

Hammer toe, floppy toe deformity and, 663
Hard callus, in bone formation, 624
Hematoma, following tibial bone grafting in foot and ankle arthrodesis, 555
    in bone formation, 624–625
Host factors, of mesenchymal stem cell grafts, 613–614
Humanitarian Device Exemption (HDE), 635

I

Iliac crest grafts. See *Autologous iliac crest bone graft (AICBG).*
Imaging, for shock wave therapy targeting, 654–657
Immobilization, following tibial bone grafting in foot and ankle arthrodesis, 557
    for stress fractures, 658
Immunomodulatory cytokines, in injured tissue, 612–613

Infection, following tibial bone grafting in foot and ankle arthrodesis, 555
   recombinant human BMP-2 and, 586, 595
   synthetic bone grafts and, 559, 563
   with fractures, autologous bone grafts and, 598–599, 604
      bone morphogenetic proteins for, retrospective review of, 545–546
      stem cell grafting and, 611
Inflammation, in bone formation, 624–625
Insulinlike growth factor (IGF), bone healing function of, 642
IntegraOS product, 614, 617
Internal fixation, in floppy toe surgery, 665–667
   of osteoporotic ankle fractures, calcium sulfate grafts for, 563–567
   open reduction and, of calcaneal fractures, calcium phosphate grafts for, 568
   tissue engineering and, 544
Interphalangeal joint, proximal, bone block lengthening of, for floppy toe deformity,
   663–668. See also *Proximal interphalangeal (PIP) joint.*
Intramedullary nail (IMN) fixation, for long bone nonunion, 604
   for tibial fractures, autologous bone grafts with, 598–600
      bone morphogenetic proteins used with, 546–547, 578, 601
Isoform/isotypes, of platelet-derived growth factor, 623–624
Italian Observational Study (BIOS) Group, on BMP-7, 601–602

   K

Kirschner wire fixation, in floppy toe surgery, 665–667

   L

Low-intensity pulsed ultrasonography (LIPUS), for stress fractures, 658
Lumbar fusion, autologous iliac crest bone graft for, 603–604
   recombinant human BMP-7 for, 602–603

   M

Macrophages, in bone formation, 624
   platelet-derived growth factors expression by, 623
Marketing, of bone graft substitutes, 560
Matrices. See *Bone matrix/matrices.*
Medical Device Amendment (1976), 560
Megakaryocytes, platelet-derived growth factors expression by, 623
Mesenchymal stem cells (MSCs), bone formation function of, 612, 623–624
   immunomodulatory characteristics of, 612
   in bone grafting, **611–619**
      advances in, 611
      as allograft, 612–613
      beta-tricalcium phosphate/collagen vs., 614–617
      culture-expanded, 612
      handling of graft, 612–613
      in humans, 612
      rationale for, 613
      suitable usage of, 614
      summary overview of, 618
      Trinity Evolution allograft and, 611–612

xenograft source of, 612
in osteoinduction, 544, 577
platelet-derived growth factors expression by, 623
tendonogenic differentiation of, 549
tissue engineering and, 544, 611–612
Messenger RNA (mRNA), sequential expression of BMP, in bone formation, 625–626
sequential expression of PDGF, in bone formation, 625
shock wave therapy impact on, 653
Metatarsophalangeal (MP) joint, in floppy toe deformity, 663–664
surgical technique consideration of, 665, 667
Mitogenesis, in bone formation, 624, 626, 628
Mozaic product, 616
Musculoskeletal repair, recombinant human platelet-derived growth factor for, **621–640**.
See also *Recombinant human platelet-derived growth factor (rhPDGF-BB)*.
Myoblasts, platelet-derived growth factors expression by, 623

N

Nail fixation. See *Intramedullary nail (IMN) fixation*.
Nanotechnology, tissue engineering role of, 547
Neovascularity. See *Angiogenesis*.
Nerve damage, autogenous bone grafts and, 559
following tibial bone grafting in foot and ankle arthrodesis, 555–556
Neurons, platelet-derived growth factors expression by, 623
Nonunion, of fractures, autologous bone grafts for, 559, 577, 597
from iliac crest, 598–602
with growth factors, 599–603
without growth factors, 598–600
bone morphogenetic proteins for, in adverse scenarios, 601–605
increased use of, 546–547, 578
initial experimental work on, 599–601
retrospective review of, 545–546, 578
platelet-rich plasma for, **641–649**. See also *Platelet-rich plasma (PRP)*.
reaming by-products for, 598–600, 604
shock wave therapy for, complications of, 656
procedure for, 655
results of, 655–656
trends of, 651–652, 654–655
stem cell grafting for, **611–619**. See also *Mesenchymal stem cells (MSCs)*.
synthetic bone grafts for. See *Synthetic bone grafts/grafting*.
tibial bone grafting for, 555
tissue engineering for, 544–545
Norian skeletal repair system (STS), 564–566, 568
North American pivotal trial, prospective 434-patient, on recombinant human
platelet-derived growth factor, 634–635
discussion on, 635–636

O

Open bone technique, for platelet-rich plasma dispensing, 645–646
Open reduction and internal fixation (ORIF), of calcaneal fractures, calcium phosphate
grafts for, 568

Orthobiologic agents, for bone healing, 545, 560
   host-surgical site indications for, 647
  for musculoskeletal repair, recombinant human platelet-derived growth factor as,
    621–640. See also *Recombinant human platelet-derived growth factor (rhPDGF-BB)*.
Osteoblasts, in bone formation, 624
  platelet-derived growth factors expression by, 623
Osteoconduction, of bone grafts, 544, 553, 559–560
Osteoconductive agents, examples of, 544, 611. See also *specific bone substitute, e.g.,*
  Calcium sulfate.
  for fracture or fusion stabilization, 579, 604
  mechanism of action, 560, 597–598
Osteoconductors, for bone healing, 577–578
   recombinant human BMP-2 use and, 594–595
Osteocytes, shock wave therapy impact on, 654
Osteogenesis, 544–545
  autologous graft material for, 553, 604. See also *Bone grafts/grafting.*
  living cells for inducing, 611–612. See also *Mesenchymal stem cells (MSCs).*
Osteogenic protein-1 (OP-1). See *Recombinant human osteogenic protein-1 (rhOP-1).*
Osteoinduction, bone healing and, 577–578
  in bone formation, 544–545
  in bone grafts, 553
Osteoinductive agents, bone morphogenetic proteins as, 577–578
   autologous bone grafts vs., 604–605
   gene technology for manufacturing, 578, 599–600
  examples of, 544–545, 598, 611
Osteoinductive matrix, as synthetic bone grafts, 560
   plus calcium phosphate, 570–571
Osteonecrosis, bone morphogenetic proteins for, 545
Osteoporosis, ankle fractures related to, calcium sulfate grafts for, 563–567
Osteoprogenitor cells, 560, 604, 612–613
  grafts of. See *Mesenchymal stem cells (MSCs).*
  in bone formation, 623–625
Osteotome, for tibial autologous graft harvest, 555, 557
Osteotomies, of metatarsals, for floppy toe correction, 665
Oxidative damage, mesenchymal stem cell grafts and, 613

P

Pain, following tibial bone grafting in foot and ankle arthrodesis, 555
Parathyroid hormone, bone healing and, 598
Percutaneous bone technique, for bone morphogenetic protein administration, 604
  for platelet-rich plasma dispensing, 646
Pericytes, 612
  platelet-derived growth factors expression by, 623
Phalanx, middle vs. proximal, in bone block lengthening of proximal interphalangeal joint for
  floppy toe deformity, 665–667
Physics, in tissue engineering, 543
PLAGA matrix, for bone morphogenetic proteins, 547–548
Platelet poor plasma (PPP), from bone marrow aspiration, 616
  wound healing properties of, 617
Platelet-derived growth factors (PDGF), basic science of, 623

bone formation role of, 623–625
    mechanism of action, 625–627
family of, 623
for musculoskeletal repair, **621–640**. See also *Recombinant human platelet-derived growth factor (rhPDGF-BB)*.
in platelet-rich plasma, 641
    bone healing function of, 598, 642–643
    concentrating system for, 647
isomer/receptor binding specificity of, 623–624
normal cell types expressing, 623
Platelet-rich plasma (PRP), for bone fusion augmentation, **641–649**
    appropriate candidates for, 646–647
    basic science of, 642–643
    bone techniques for dispensing, 645–646
    complications of, 644
    evidence-based medicine on, 643–645
    from bone marrow aspiration, 616
    growth factors in, 641–643
        concentrating system for, 647
    poor bone healing indications for, 641–642
    practical clinical considerations of, 647–648
    summary overview of, 641, 648
Platelets, platelet-derived growth factors expression by, 623
Polylactic-co-glycolic acid (PLAGA), bone healing applications of, bone morphogenetic proteins and, 547–548
Polymers, as synthetic bone grafts, 560
    plus calcium phosphate plus recombinant human bone morphogenetic protein, 571
Polymethylmethacrylate (PMMA), composite bone grafts vs., 570
    for calcaneal fractures, 567
Polyphosphazene (PPHOA) polymers, bone healing applications of, bone morphogenetic proteins and, 547
Pro-osteogenic graft materials. See *Synthetic bone grafts/grafting*.
Pro-Osteon, for backfilling, in proximal tibial autologous graft harvest, 556
Prospective 60-patient open-label Canadian registration trial, on recombinant human platelet-derived growth factor, 631–632
    discussion on, 635–636
Prospective 434-patient North American pivotal trial, on recombinant human platelet-derived growth factor, 634–635
    discussion on, 635–636
Prospective randomized controlled 20-patient US pilot trial, on recombinant human platelet-derived growth factor, 632–634
    discussion on, 635–636
Proteins, for bone formation in surgery. See *Bone morphogenetic proteins (BMPs)*.
    upregulation of, shock wave therapy impact on, 653–654
Proximal interphalangeal (PIP) joint, arthrodesis of, for flail toe, 664
    bone block lengthening of, for floppy toe deformity, **663–668**
        description of, 663–664
        summary overview of, 667
        surgical technique for, 665–667
        surgical treatment alternatives vs., 664–665
    resection arthroplasty of, for floppy toe deformity, 663–665

Proximal tibial bone grafts, for foot and ankle procedures, 554–556
  authors' preferred harvest technique for, 555–556
 thumb-distance incision for harvest of, 555–556

  R

Raynaud disease, flail toe deformity and, 664
Reactive oxygen species (ROS), mesenchymal stem cell grafts and, 613
Reaming by-products (RBP), for fracture management, 598–600, 604
Receptor binding specificity, of platelet-derived growth factor, 623–624
Recombinant gene technology, for manufacturing osteoinductive proteins, 578, 599–600
Recombinant human BMP-2 (rhBMP-2), for bone healing, **577–596**
  FDA approval of, 578
  gene technology for manufacturing, 578, 599–600
  initial experimental work on, 599–601
  physiologic mechanisms of, 577–578
  plus calcium phosphate and polymers, 571
  retrospective studies and reviews of, 545–546, 578
   material and methods for, 578–579
   overall results, 579
   patient categorization for, 579
   tibia/ankle/foot results, 579, 583–585
    average time to healing, 583
    case presentation of ankle, 586, 589–591
    case presentation of foot, 587–588, 592–594
    case presentation of tibia, 586–588
    determination of time to healing, 583
    discussion on, 588–595
    patient database of, 580–585
    segmental tibial bone loss example, 583, 585
    subtalar fusion example, 583, 585, 593
    talonavicular fusion example, 583–584
    used alone vs. with adjuncts, 583, 585
Recombinant human BMP-7 (rhBMP-7). See also *Recombinant human osteogenic protein-1 (rhOP-1).*
  for bone healing, 577–578
   cost considerations of, 605
   efficacy and safety of, 601–603
   in adverse scenarios, 604–605
   retrospective studies and reviews of, 545–546, 589, 600
   with autologous bone grafts, initial experimental work on, 600–601
    observational studies of, 601–603
  for spinal fusion, 602–603
Recombinant human bone morphogenetic protein. See also *Recombinant human BMP entries.*
  as synthetic bone grafts, plus calcium phosphate and polymers, 571
Recombinant human osteogenic protein-1 (rhOP-1), for bone healing. See also *Recombinant human BMP-7 (rhBMP-7).*
  FDA approval of, 546–547
  initial experimental work on, 600–601
  PLAGA matrix and, 547–548

with autologous bone grafts, 578, 589, 601
    in adverse scenarios, 601–603
Recombinant human platelet-derived growth factor (rhPDGF-BB), for foot and ankle fusion,
   621–640
    autogenous bone grafts vs., 621–622
    development of, animal research in, 630–631
       human studies in, 627–630
       sequential stringent studies in, 636
       technology for, 622–623, 627
    discussion on, 635–636
    efficacy and safety of, 635–636
    FDA approval of, 632, 635–636
    future expanded role of, 636
    prospective 60-patient open-label Canadian registration trial on, 631–632
    prospective 434-patient North American pivotal trial on, 634–635
    prospective randomized controlled 20-patient US pilot trial on, 632–634
Regranex gel, as recombinant human platelet-derived growth factor, 628–629
Regulation, of β-tricalcium phosphate/collagen, 614
   of bone graft substitutes, 560
   of recombinant human BMP-2, 578
   of recombinant human osteogenic protein-1, 546–547
   of recombinant human platelet-derived growth factor, 632, 635–636
   of shock wave therapy applications, 652
Rehabilitation, following tibial bone grafting in foot and ankle arthrodesis, 555
Remodeling, in bone formation, 624–625
Resection arthroplasty, of proximal interphalangeal joint, for floppy toe deformity, 663–665
rhBMP2 Infuse Bonegraft. See Recombinant human BMP-2 (rhBMP-2).

S

Safety, of recombinant human BMP-7, 601–603
   of recombinant human platelet-derived growth factor, 635–636
Salvage procedures, recombinant human BMP-2 used with, 593–594
   tissue engineering and, 545
Scaffold material, bone grafts and, 560, 597
   in bone healing, 577
   in tissue engineering, 544
      bone morphogenetic proteins and, 547–549
   recombinant human platelet-derived growth factor combined with, 622, 630
   stem cell grafts and, 611
Screw fixation, tibia pro fibular, of osteoporotic ankle fractures, calcium sulfate grafts for,
   563–567
Segmental bone loss, bone morphogenetic proteins for, 545, 604
   mesenchymal stem cell grafts for, 613
   tibial, recombinant human BMP-2 for, 583, 585
      recombinant human osteogenic protein-1 for, 601
Sensory loss, following tibial bone grafting in foot and ankle arthrodesis, 555
Serotonin (5HT), bone healing function of, 642
Shock wave generators, 652
Shock wave therapy (SWT), for bone pathology, **651–662**
      avascular necrosis as, 651–652, 656–657

Shock wave therapy (*continued*)
  basic principles of, 652
  biologic response to, 653–654
  clinical focusing of, 654
  FDA approval of, 652
  high- vs. low-energy, 652–653
  nonunion as, 651, 654–656
  parameters for, 652–653
  procedures for, 654–658
    general considerations of, 654
    specific bone disorders, 654–658
  stress fractures as, 651, 657–658
  summary overview of, 658
  trends of, 651–652
Shock waves, direct vs. indirect effect on tissues, 652
    biologic responses to, 653–654
  physical properties of, 652
  production devices for, 652
  radial, 652
Short floppy toe deformity, description of, 663–664
  surgical management of, **663–668**. See also *Bone block lengthening.*
Skeletal repair system (STS), Norian, 564–566
Smooth muscle cells, vascular, platelet-derived growth factors expression by, 623
Soft callus, in bone formation, 624
Soft tissue injuries, bone morphogenetic proteins for, 548–549
  graft docking site and, 604–605
  shock wave therapy for, 651–652
  tissue engineering for, 544
Spinal surgery. See also *Lumbar fusion.*
  bone morphogenetic proteins in, 545
Sponge application technique, for recombinant human BMP-7, 591–592
Stem cells, as grafts. See *Mesenchymal stem cells (MSCs).*
  recruitment of, shock wave therapy impact on, 653
Stress fractures, following tibial bone grafting in foot and ankle arthrodesis, 557
  shock wave therapy for, 651, 657–658
Subtalar fusion, recombinant human BMP-2 used in, 583, 585, 593
Syndactylization, for flail toe correction, 664
Synthetic bone grafts/grafting, **559–576**
  calcium phosphate as, 560, 563–568
    plus calcium sulfate, 569
    plus osteoinductive matrix, 570–571
    plus recombinant human bone morphogenetic protein plus polymers, 571
  calcium sulfate as, 560–563
    plus calcium phosphate, 569
  composite, 569–571
  osteoinductive matrix as, plus calcium phosphate, 570–571
  platelet-rich plasma used with, 647–648
  polymers as, 560
    plus calcium phosphate plus recombinant human bone morphogenetic protein, 571
  recombinant human bone morphogenetic protein as, plus calcium phosphate and
    polymers, 571

summary overview of, 571
TCP as. See *Tricalcium phosphate (TCP)*.

T

Talonavicular fusion, recombinant human BMP-2 used in, 583–584
Template, in tissue engineering, 544
Tendon lengthening, in floppy toe surgery, 665
Tendon repair, growth/differentiation factors for, 548–549
Thrombospondin-1, bone healing function of, 642
Tibia pro fibular screw fixation, of osteoporotic ankle fractures, calcium sulfate grafts for, 563–567
Tibial bone grafts, for foot and ankle procedures, **553–558**
     advantages of, 554
     distal, 556–557
          authors' preferred harvest technique for, 557
          medial incision for harvest of, 557
     proximal, 554–556
          authors' preferred harvest technique for, 555–556
          thumb-distance incision for harvest of, 555–556
     reaming by-products and, 598–600, 604
     summary overview of, 557
Tibial fractures, autologous bone grafts for, with growth factors, 598–603
     with intramedullary nail fixation, 598–601
     without growth factors, 598–600
   bone morphogenetic proteins for, complications of, 547
     recombinant human BMP-2 studies of, 579, 583–585
          average time to healing, 583
          case presentation of, 586–588
          case presentation of ankle vs., 586, 589–591
          case presentation of foot vs., 587–588, 592–594
          comorbidities and, 595
          complications of, 592–593
          cost considerations of, 589–591, 605
          determination of time to healing, 583
          discussion on, 588–595
          further research on, 595
          osteoconductor indications with, 594–595
          overall results vs., 579
          patient database of, 580–585
          patient risk level and, 593
          salvage procedures and, 593–594
          segmental bone loss example, 583, 585, 601
          sponge application technique in, 591–592
          subtalar fusion example vs., 583, 585, 593
          talonavicular fusion example vs., 583–584
          uniqueness of, 589
          used alone vs. with adjuncts, 583, 585
     studies of, 546–547, 578–579
     with intramedullary nail fixation, 546–547, 578, 601
   intramedullary nail fixation for, autologous bone grafts with, 598–603

Tibial fractures (*continued*)
    bone morphogenetic proteins with, 546–547, 578, 601
    reaming by-products for, 598–600, 604
Time to healing, in tibial/ankle/foot conditions, 583
Tissue engineering, beta-tricalcium phosphate/collagen in, 614–618
    bone morphogenetic proteins for, 543–547
        clinical indications and outcomes in, 544
            recent studies of, 545–546
            retrospective review of, 545–546
        complications associated with, 547
        electrospinning and, 547
        fixation devices and, 545
        future trends for, 547–549
        in foot and ankle surgery, **577–596**. See also *Recombinant human BMP-2 (rhBMP-2); Recombinant human BMP-7 (rhBMP-7)*.
        in fracture care, 546
            for nonunion repair, 546–547
        in soft tissue repair, 548–549
        initial description of, 545
        mechanism of action, 545
        methods for incorporation of, 545
        natural healing process vs., 544
        osteoconduction and, 544
        osteoinduction and, 544–545
        polylactic-co-glycolic acid vs., 547–548
        polyphosphazene polymers vs., 547
        summary overview of, 549
    definition of, 543–544
    in surgery, advances in, 543–544, 549
        clinical indications and outcomes of, 544
    nanotechnology role in, 547
    stem cell grafts in, 611–614, 618. See also *Mesenchymal stem cells (MSCs)*.
Total ankle replacement (TAR), Agility, platelet-rich plasma for, 644–645
Transforming growth factor β (TGF-β), bone healing function of, 642–643
    bone morphogenetic proteins as, 577. See also *Bone morphogenetic proteins (BMPs)*.
    tissue engineering and, 545
Trauma management. See also *Fractures*.
    bone morphogenetic proteins in, 545
        autologous bone grafts vs., 604–605
    calcium phosphate grafts for, 567–568
Tricalcium phosphate (TCP). See also *β-Tricalcium phosphate (β-TCP)/collagen*.
    as synthetic bone grafts, 560, 569–570, 579
Trinity Evolution allograft, augmentation properties of, 612
    evolution of, 611–612
    handling of, 612–613
    mesenchymal stem cells vs., 612–613
    rationale behind, 613
    suitable usage of, 614
Trocar, for bone marrow harvest between iliac walls, 615–616

U

Ultrasonography, for shock wave therapy targeting, 654–657
    low-intensity pulsed, for stress fractures, 658
    tissue engineering and, 544
Union, of fractures. See *Nonunion.*
US pilot trial, prospective randomized controlled 20-patient, on recombinant human
    platelet-derived growth factor, 632–634
            discussion on, 635–636

V

Vascular endothelial growth (VEGF), 623
    bone healing function of, 642–643
    shock wave therapy impact on, 653
Vascular smooth muscle cells, platelet-derived growth factors expression by, 623
Vitoss product, 614

W

Weight bearing, postoperative, in bone block lengthening of proximal interphalangeal
    joint for floppy toe deformity, 667
        in tibial bone grafting in foot and ankle arthrodesis, 555, 557
        stress fractures and, 658
Wire fixation, Kirschner, in floppy toe surgery, 665–667
Wound closure, in proximal tibial autologous graft harvest, 555
Wound healing, platelet poor plasma for, 617
    recombinant human platelet-derived growth factor for, 628

X

Xenograft-sourced mesenchymal stem cells, 612

Y

Yeast expression system, for recombinant human platelet-derived growth factor
    production, 627–628

Z

Zones of injury, 612

United States Postal Service

Statement of Ownership, Management, and Circulation
(All Periodicals Publications Except Requestor Publications)

1. Publication Title	2. Publication Number	3. Filing Date
Foot and Ankle Clinics	0 1 6 - 3 6 8	9/15/10

4. Issue Frequency	5. Number of Issues Published Annually	6. Annual Subscription Price
Mar, Jun, Sep, Dec	4	$253.00

7. Complete Mailing Address of Known Office of Publication (Not printer) (Street, city, county, state, and ZIP+4®)

Elsevier Inc.
360 Park Avenue South
New York, NY 10010-1710

Contact Person
Stephen Bushing
Telephone (Include area code)
215-239-3688

8. Complete Mailing Address of Headquarters or General Business Office of Publisher (Not printer)

Elsevier Inc., 360 Park Avenue South, New York, NY 10010-1710

9. Full Names and Complete Mailing Addresses of Publisher, Editor, and Managing Editor (Do not leave blank)

Publisher (Name and complete mailing address)

Kim Murphy, Elsevier, Inc., 1600 John F. Kennedy Blvd. Suite 1800, Philadelphia, PA 19103-2899

Editor (Name and complete mailing address)

Deb Dellapena, Elsevier, Inc., 1600 John F. Kennedy Blvd. Suite 1800, Philadelphia, PA 19103-2899

Managing Editor (Name and complete mailing address)

Catherine Bewick, Elsevier, Inc., 1600 John F. Kennedy Blvd. Suite 1800, Philadelphia, PA 19103-2899

10. Owner (Do not leave blank. If the publication is owned by a corporation, give the name and address of the corporation immediately followed by the names and addresses of all stockholders owning or holding 1 percent or more of the total amount of stock. If not owned by a corporation, give the names and addresses of the individual owners. If owned by a partnership or other unincorporated firm, give its name and address as well as those of each individual owner. If the publication is published by a nonprofit organization, give its name and address.)

Full Name	Complete Mailing Address
Wholly owned subsidiary of	4520 East-West Highway
Reed/Elsevier, US holdings	Bethesda, MD 20814

11. Known Bondholders, Mortgagees, and Other Security Holders Owning or Holding 1 Percent or More of Total Amount of Bonds, Mortgages, or Other Securities. If none, check box. ☐ None

Full Name	Complete Mailing Address
N/A	

12. Tax Status (For completion by nonprofit organizations authorized to mail at nonprofit rates) (Check one)
The purpose, function, and nonprofit status of this organization and the exempt status for federal income tax purposes:
☐ Has Not Changed During Preceding 12 Months
☐ Has Changed During Preceding 12 Months (Publisher must submit explanation of change with this statement)

PS Form 3526, September 2007 (Page 1 of 3 (Instructions Page 3)) PSN 7530-01-000-9931 PRIVACY NOTICE: See our Privacy policy in www.usps.com

---

13. Publication Title		14. Issue Date for Circulation Data Below
Foot and Ankle Clinics		September 2010

15. Extent and Nature of Circulation			Average No. Copies Each Issue During Preceding 12 Months	No. Copies of Single Issue Published Nearest to Filing Date
a. Total Number of Copies (Net press run)			1426	1414
b. Paid Circulation (By Mail and Outside the Mail)	(1)	Mailed Outside-County Paid Subscriptions Stated on PS Form 3541. (Include paid distribution above nominal rate, advertiser's proof copies, and exchange copies)	786	748
	(2)	Mailed In-County Paid Subscriptions Stated on PS Form 3541 (Include paid distribution above nominal rate, advertiser's proof copies, and exchange copies)		
	(3)	Paid Distribution Outside the Mails Including Sales Through Dealers and Carriers, Street Vendors, Counter Sales, and Other Paid Distribution Outside USPS®	171	165
	(4)	Paid Distribution by Other Classes Mailed Through the USPS (e.g. First-Class Mail®)		
c. Total Paid Distribution (Sum of 15b (1), (2), (3), and (4))		▶	957	913
d. Free or Nominal Rate Distribution (By Mail and Outside the Mail)	(1)	Free or Nominal Rate Outside-County Copies Included on PS Form 3541	61	24
	(2)	Free or Nominal Rate In-County Copies Included on PS Form 3541		
	(3)	Free or Nominal Rate Copies Mailed at Other Classes Through the USPS (e.g. First-Class Mail)		
	(4)	Free or Nominal Rate Distribution Outside the Mail (Carriers or other means)		
e. Total Free or Nominal Rate Distribution (Sum of 15d (1), (2), (3) and (4))		▶	61	24
f. Total Distribution (Sum of 15c and 15e)		▶	1018	937
g. Copies not Distributed (See instructions to publishers #4 (page #3))		▶	408	477
h. Total (Sum of 15f and g)		▶	1426	1414
i. Percent Paid (15c divided by 15f times 100)			94.01%	97.44%

16. Publication of Statement of Ownership

☑ If the publication is a general publication, publication of this statement is required. Will be printed in the **December 2010** issue of this publication. ☐ Publication not required

17. Signature and Title of Editor, Publisher, Business Manager, or Owner	Date
[signature] Stephen R. Bushing – Fulfillment/Inventory Specialist	September 15, 2010

I certify that all information furnished on this form is true and complete. I understand that anyone who furnishes false or misleading information on this form or who omits material or information requested on the form may be subject to criminal sanctions (including fines and imprisonment) and/or civil sanctions (including civil penalties).

PS Form 3526, September 2007 (Page 2 of 3)

Moving?

Make sure your subscription moves with you!

To notify us of your new address, find your **Clinics Account Number** (located on your mailing label above your name), and contact customer service at:

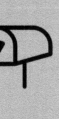

Email: journalscustomerservice-usa@elsevier.com

800-654-2452 (subscribers in the U.S. & Canada)
314-447-8871 (subscribers outside of the U.S. & Canada)

Fax number: 314-447-8029

Elsevier Health Sciences Division
Subscription Customer Service
3251 Riverport Lane
Maryland Heights, MO 63043

Printed and bound by CPI Group (UK) Ltd, Croydon, CR0 4YY

03/10/2024

01040445-0013